Foraged Condiments

Foraged Condiments

Wild Plant Recipes for Sauces, Chutneys, Ferments and Drinks

Natasha Lloyd

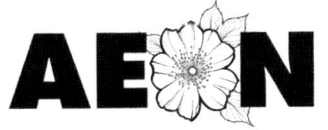

First published in 2025 by
Aeon Books

Copyright ©2025 by Natasha Lloyd
Plant portraits ©2025 by Ashley Cook

The right of Natasha Lloyd to be identified as the author of this work has been asserted in accordance with §§77 and 78 of the Copyright Design and Patents Act 1988.

All rights reserved. No part of this publication may be reproduced, stored in a retrieval system, or transmitted, in any form or by any means, electronic, mechanical, photocopying, recording, or otherwise, without the prior written permission of the publisher.

British Cataloguing in Publication Data
A C.I.P. for this book is available from the British Library

ISBN-13: 978-1-91280-798-7

Edited by Matthew Seal
Typesetting and design by Julie Bruton-Seal
Printed and bound by Short Run Press Ltd, Exeter EX2 7LW

www.aeonbooks.co.uk

Disclaimer
The content of this book is for information purposes and not a substitute for professional medical advice, diagnosis or treatment. It does not contribute to health advice. Consult with your doctor or another healthcare professional like a medical herbalist for medical conditions. I take no responsibility for a person foraging for plants or fungi, which if done incorrectly can result in injury, harm and even death.

Dedication

To Mum, Dad, my brother Ollie, Rosie dog, Yarrow dog, Chammy pup and Dandelion cat.

With thanks to:

Ashley Cook for the beautiful plant illustrations.
Amy Muir for the outside photos.
Thank you to Sam Webster for the photo of fermented wild garlic.
With thanks and gratitude to Rachel and Layla for their support and love.
Anne Campbell for the Gaelic names of the plants.
To one particular friend who listened extensively and allowed me to bounce ideas and thoughts, thank you for your logical mind and your time.
Thanks to Greg Powers for the handmade bowls kindly gifted. They can be purchased at the Durslade Farm Shop and in Mayfair Farm Shop. Also on his website www.blightybushcraft.co.uk
Thanks to Rob for picking me up while hitchhiking and all your support in the kitchen and beyond.
Thanks to Iwan and Manuela for taking a risk on a random hitchhiker and your support and kindness.
Thanks to Vivienne Campbell for her encouragement and love at the very beginning of this project.
Thanks to the team at Aeon: without your support and long patience this book wouldn't be here.
A heartfelt thanks to you all.

Contents

Introduction 9

Foraging   11

Plants   29
Bogbean 31   Bramble 35   Common hogweed 39   Dandelion 45
Elderberry 49   Ground Elder 53   Hawthorn 57   Jack by the hedge 63
Nettle 69   Pineapple mayweed 73   Plantain 75   Rosebay willowherb 79
Rowan or mountain ash 83   Scots pine 87   Silver birch 91
Sweet cicely 95   Valerian 99   Wild garlic 103   Wild raspberry 107
Yarrow 111

Recipes   115
Dipping sauces 117   Chutneys 121   Ferments 127   Jams and jellies 131
Aiolis and pestos 139   Salad dressings 143   Salts and a sugar 147
Ketchups 153   Sauces, stuffings and a coating 155 Vinegars 159
Pickles 161   Hot drinks and a rob 165   Tonic waters 173   Vermouths 179
Syrups 183 Turkish delights 189   Bitters 193

Wild food diary   197

Bibliography 219

Index 221

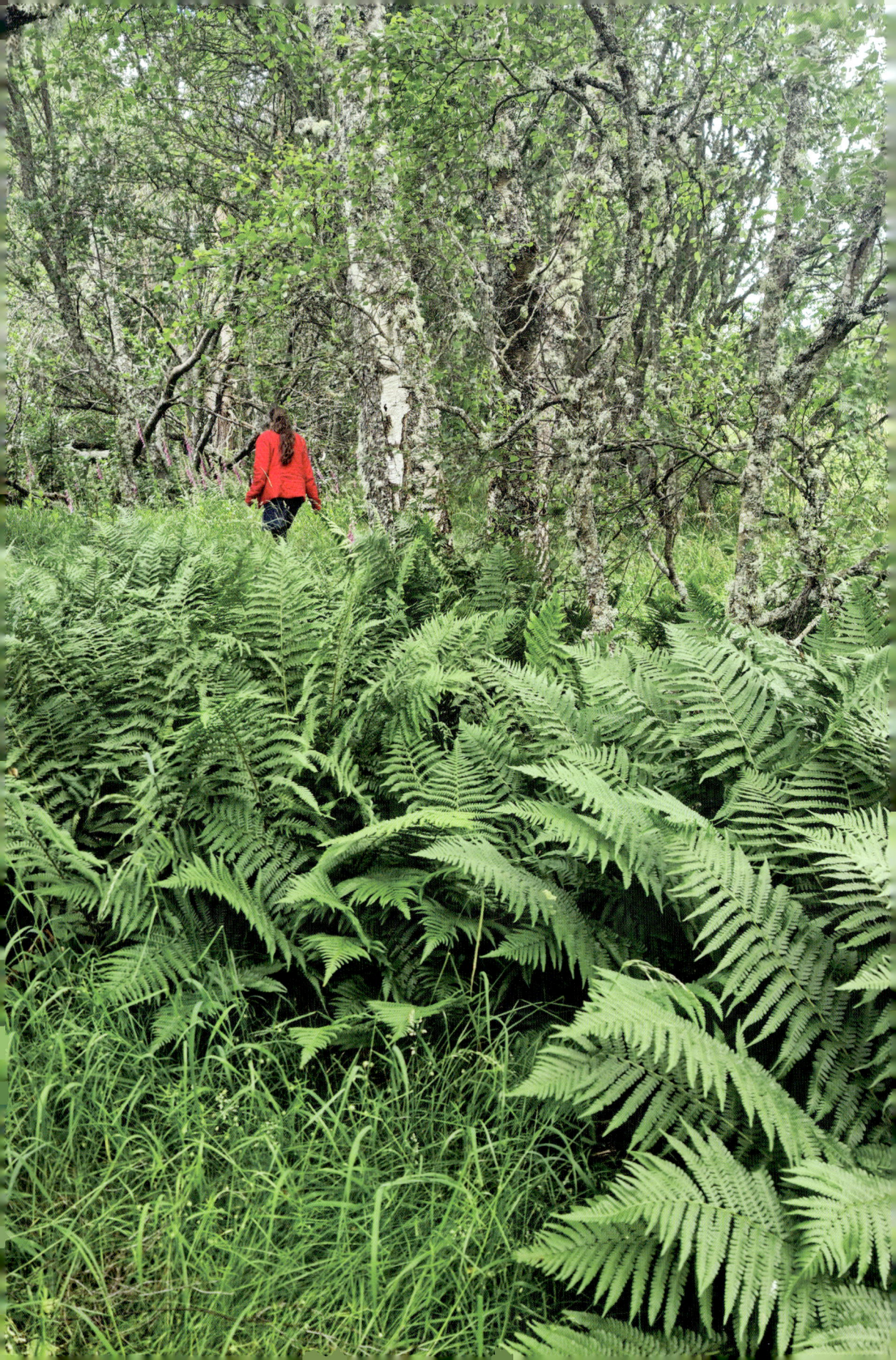

Introduction

Choosing the plants included in this book was easy as they grow locally to me and are familiar. The hard part was limiting it to just twenty. I know them well, love them and wanted to present them to with a wider knowledge than I can do on a walk or workshop. We would be there all day on a few plants otherwise. The walks are for an introduction to the fascinating world of plants, foraging and learning on how to connect to nature.

Originally I saw Ashley Cook's work at The Braemar Gallery and felt very drawn to her work. It is rare that a piece of art draws me in to this extent. One Saturday evening I plucked up courage to email Ashley and ask if she had availability and would she be interested. To my delight she did and was interested. We worked out a time which worked for both of us. I would spend time sitting with the plants and thinking about them. Then I would convey this to Ashley and she came up with the beautiful illustrations. I was amazed at seeing the thoughts and words becoming artwork. We resonated so well it was a great joy to work with Ashley as she conveyed so well what was in my thoughts. A very impressive skill. It was all about connection to the plants and with each other.

Choosing the recipes was a joy in itself. After working in The Fife Arms kitchen creating condiments for the hotel I gained a lot of knowledge and confidence. I worked with some fantastic chefs and there was a buzz in the kitchen. I love food and flavours, so adding the skills to help these develop in the mouth took the results to another level. I have kept it simple in this book so you can experience the flavours of nature yourself with only the equipment you probably already have in your kitchen. I hope you enjoy them.

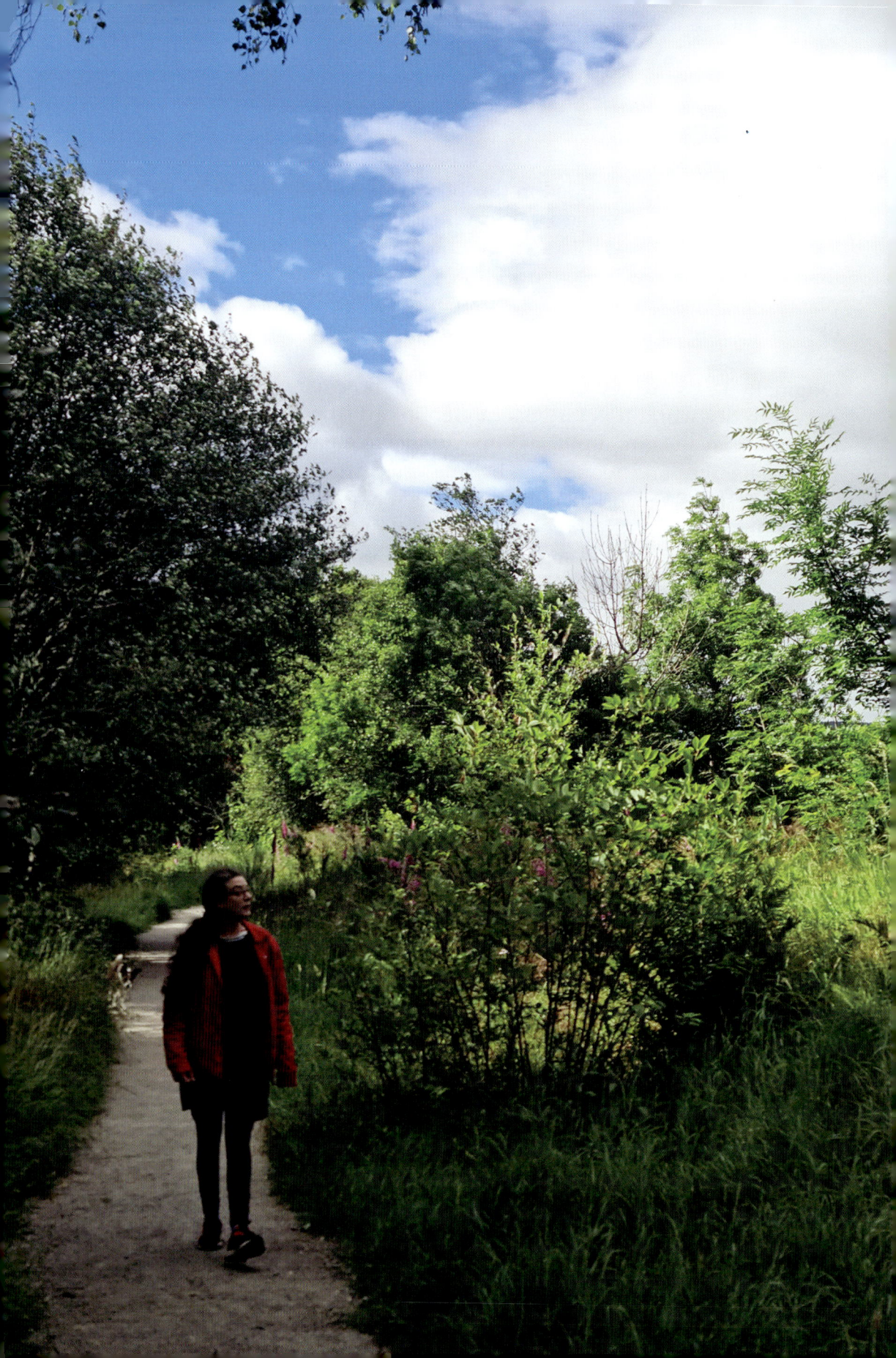

Foraging

As a child I was often outside. My Mum would take us bramble picking in the Autumn, and we would discuss the plants we saw. How long has this bush been here? How old is it and is it older than the bush we see? Does it like its plant neighbours? Who would have picked from here in the past? Questions and thoughts like these allowed a young mind to wander and think.

I remember the day I was weeding the front garden. We lived in a block of flats at the time, and keeping your front garden was important because it meant the estate looked good. At times it was more of a chore than a joy for me as a young girl. We were not the 'keeping up appearances' type and I didn't see the point in it. At this age I was unaware of neighbourly and societal pressure, but my Mum was often asking me to weed the garden.

I became annoyed one day and didn't want to continue my task. I suddenly had questions. Why does this plant get to live here but this one doesn't? I found it harder and harder to pull out the young plants – surely they deserved a chance at life too! My Mum explained the details of nutrients and space for the plants to grow and said that pulling up the young nettles would help the other plants have their own space and nutrients. She went on to say if we looked elsewhere, locally, we would find that plant growing. So she took me to the local nettle patch on a patch of waste ground nearby.

Mum saw my interest, concern and connection with the plants and took me inside. She showed me a copy of Mrs Grieve's book *A Modern Herbal* (1931), and we looked up a few plants. That day I found my passion for plants and especially for weeds, the plants considered to be in the wrong place. For the next few years of that garden I would find a weed in the waste ground, ask Mum what it was, and look it up the book. I still use that book today. So for me foraging and plants have always been a part of life. Then I followed my passion and went on to train as a medical herbalist. A lot of the plants I knew as a child I now use in practice.

When I was growing up my Mum told me we are related to the Beaton family, a clan with a strong medical tradition (see John Bannerman, *The Beatons: A*

Medical Kindred in the Classical Gaelic Tradition, 1998). At the time I didn't think much of the connection and almost dismissed it. Then, when researching for my dissertation, I learnt more about the Beatons, and now wonder how much of my love and passion for herbal medicine and foraging is in the blood. I have a natural passion for plants and nature, and my ancestors did so too as their role in their communities. So it's perfectly natural that I would do this in my community too.

Foraging, hunting and gathering

We have foraged for thousands of years. It is natural and instinctual to us. In a sense we still do it on a daily basis – it is just that we now use supermarkets, local suppliers and online resources. For most things shopping is a simple process of choosing what we want and ordering it. Say, for example, I want baked beans, then I ask what brand do I prefer? Do I want them spiced up or flavoured? What is available and is anything on offer?

When it comes to fruit and vegetables it is a slightly more in-depth process as they are fresh. We look, feel and smell for their freshness and for any signs of deterioration. In our modern ways we also check the best-before dates, but really we use more of our senses to see if they are as fresh as possible. We look carefully, and quite often folk will pick up a fruit or vegetable and give it a squeeze and quick sniff – not always socially acceptable these days. All these factors all give us information to decide if this is a good item to take home and use.

The use of plastic coverings for fruit and veg has created a distance between us and them. Some folk would say it's for the better. It is more convenient to the customer, there are fewer issues with contamination, it is easier to deal with at the checkout and easier to transport.

We still instinctively scan our fresh produce for signs of deterioration. We also know where most items we are looking for are located in a shop, because there is a planned format to most shops, with bread in one area, milk and chilled goods in the fridge, canned items and dry goods on a shelf.

Foraging in the wild isn't that different really, just the space in between each item is usually a bit further apart. When looking for, say, wild garlic I know it is going to be growing in semi-open woodland, so that is where I head. With a little experience of foraging you know where your patches are for your favourite foods. So we make our way to the local wild garlic patch and scan the area, looking for the familiar leaves. We head over to the patch and check more closely to see if the leaves are big enough to harvest or too old to bother with. If they are too young, we'll want to wait for them to grow a bit more, giving us a better harvest. We want the best for our dinner!

We also check to see if the plants are definitely wild garlic and not lords and ladies (*Arum maculatum*) or bluebell leaves. Both grow alongside wild garlic but neither are what you want to eat. Lords and ladies leaves are highly irritant, making your mouth smart as though you are trying to eating lots of small needles. Bluebell leaves are poisonous so must be avoided.

Now we crush and smell the leaf in front of us, and that familiar wild garlic odour hits our memory. We have identified it and can safely take it home to create delicious food for ourselves.

When foraging it is important to think about supply in a different way. The supermarkets are topped up with food more regularly than your local wild garlic patch can be. We have to learn to think about how the plant will survive into next year's growth. We need to bear in mind that the plant usually only comes up once a year. Other folk will also gather from that patch too, so only take what you need – not what you *want* but *need*, for your dinner that day.

The idea is to leave plenty behind for others in your community and any wildlife that also use it for food, along with enough for the plant to survive into next year. It is a different way of thinking, but once you start to understand it will become more natural to you, and you will start to feel the seasons and pulse of nature more acutely. A joy.

No matter how you came to foraging in our modern world you will still have some inherent ability without even knowing it. Some call it instinct, others say it is learned memory from ancient times. Tapping into that is deeply connecting, and you'll find that it is good for your mind.

Hunting and gathering go back to the beginnings of the human race. We wouldn't be here without our ancestors hunting and gathering for food. Of course, none of this was documented until much, much later. Oral traditions were the only way information was passed on until the invention of written language, ink and paper. Even then it was a time-consuming and costly activity to write. Paper and ink had to be hand-made so only what was considered important information was documented. To a degree the daily task of gathering food and hunting was so normal it wasn't even considered worthy of writing down. Unlike now where we can write easily and freely, sometimes too easily!

The knowledge of hunting animals has been found in cave art in the form of pictures, but the knowledge of plants took longer to be depicted and eventually be written down.

The Scottish connection
Some 6000 years ago Scotland was about 80% covered in forests and woodlands. These were good hunting grounds for animals but were not considered places to set up home for the night owing to the dangers that those animals posed to humans. Humans at that stage were nomadic and semi-nomadic, moving with the seasons and conditions from place to place. There is archaeological evidence that most folk stayed close to the coastlines and didn't often venture inland. This indicates there was an abundance of food for them at the sites they chose. The seas and rivers would have had plenty of fish and shellfish for human consumption.

Settling and moving away from a nomadic lifestyle seem to begin in the Mesolithic period when there is more evidence of tool- and boat-making. This enabled easier travel to hunting grounds. Charred remains of animal bones, shellfish and hazelnut husks are found in many sites. Naturally the plants used were not documented in charred remains as they turn to ash and are lost in the dust of time. Still I find it fun to speculate how plants may have been used: was a venison joint wrapped in leaves after being cooked to keep it fresh until it was eaten? A lot of plants have antimicrobial properties so it isn't too far a stretch to think the leaves may have helped preserve the meat. Speculation aside, knowledge of plants only really comes from written texts owing to the transient nature of plant matter.

We do have some evidence to show that in the Neolithic period the beginnings of agriculture featured certain cereal crops being grown, such as emmer, wheat and barley. The Bronze Age and Middle Ages saw an influx of people into Scotland. This allowed current settlements to grow and new ones to emerge. With more people joining and creating new areas for settlement society started to change, with folk taking on more defined roles within a social structure and hierarchical modes of thinking being established.

We then start to get written texts, which allow us to glean information about the uses of plants. Travelling monks and scholars are known to have been the first scribes of texts and had formal gardens to grow certain plants. Some plants were more for food and others for medicine, although most food has both medicinal and nutritional benefits. From around 400BC we have the Greek physician and philosopher Hippocrates saying 'Let food be thy medicine and medicine be thy food'.

As a medical herbalist and forager I'm acutely aware that food and medicine are intertwined and improve our health. The very act of foraging is good for us in that we get exercise and spend time outside. Then add in the freshness of the food we gather and the nutritious benefits of that food from soil without added chemicals, and it all brings benefit to us.

Modern medicine is relatively new in this context and even now, a significant number of modern drugs come from plants originally.

The written record
I will focus on Scotland in what follows primarily because I live here and it is familiar to me. There is also a clear path of the route of medicinal information about plants coming from the old Greek method of medicine. Food plants were not written down so we have to look at the medicinal plants that were recorded. Of the few Gaelic manuscripts that have been translated it is clearly Greek medicine thinking that influences these texts. There are several that haven't been translated yet, and it would be so interesting to see what is in those manuscripts.

If we go right back to the first known medicinal texts in history they come from Egypt and are written on papyrus. These include the Ramesseum Medical Papyri from around 1800 BCE, the Kahun Gynaecological Papyrus from much the same date, the London Medical Papyrus from around 1600 BCE, the Ebers Papyrus from around 1550 BCE, the Edwin Smith Papyrus from around 1500 BCE, and the Brugsch Papyrus from around 1200 BCE.

Egyptian thinking was adopted into Greek thinking, and an important collection of medical writings known as the Hippocratic Corpus was compiled between 400 BCE and 200 BCE. This included the Hippocratic oath that is still in use in medical schools today. Then came the Galenic Corpus, the work of the Greek physician and philosopher Galen of Pergamon (AD 129–216), and before this Dioscorides (AD c.40–90) wrote five volumes of *De Materia Medica*. This became the standard textbook for the Middle Ages, and mentions about 600 plants. Pliny the Elder wrote his *Naturalis Historia*, a 10-volume work, in AD 77.

The Anglo-Saxon *Book of Bald* in AD 900 makes reference to Scottish plants. With the onset of Christianity moving into Ireland and the west coast of Scotland, it was the travelling monks that brought their texts with them. It is thought it is one of these monastic texts that the Beaton family used.

In the late 1600s a famine hit the east coast of Scotland, which prompted the physician Robert Sibbald (1641–1722) to write *Provision for the Poor in time of Dearth and Scarcity* in 1699. This study of edible plants in the area is the first known foraging book and writing down of food plants. In the same year Sibbald oversaw publication of the first *Edinburgh Pharmacopoeia*. He also commissioned the writer Martin Martin (1660–1718) to go into the Highlands and the Islands to gather stories and information.

Martin published his account in 1703 under the title *A Description of The Western Isles of Scotland*. This then inspired other folk to follow, with the first systematic study of the plants of Scotland being John Lightfoot's *Flora Scotia*, published in 1777. Coming a bit more up to date, we see John Cameron's *The Gaelic Names of Plants (Scottish, Irish and Manx)* in 1883. And in 1951 the School of Scottish Studies was set up to gather and record as much as possible the stories and culture of Scotland. This is easily accessed via their website.

A few books have been published that also document uses of plants in Scotland in modern times and are worth seeking out. I've listed them in the Bibliography.

Foraging and weeding
When folk started to settle into suitable areas to live they started to grow plants around their settlements. Sometimes these were close by and sometimes further afield if it was a larger crop that needed more space. Plants and vegetables would have been grown collectively and for the benefit of the whole settlement and community. With the settling and growing of plants for food choice became more of an option. That is the beginning of gardening and horticulture. We started to choose what we grow for ourselves instead of finding and foraging what edible plants grew close by. This would also have been the beginning of weeding.

During the lockdowns I wrote a few pieces for The Fife Arms of Braemar on nature, selecting a few seasonal plants to focus on that folk could find on their walks in their local area. At that time we were restricted in our movements and people were going for more walks. One plant I chose was dandelion. I mentioned in passing how the settlers of North America took dandelion with them to grow as useful lawns. One gentleman wrote to me to challenge this idea. I understood his perspective as these days folk spend time trying to weed out and eradicate dandelion from their grass lawns.

The settlers taking dandelion to grow is not that dissimilar to hunter gatherers settling and growing what they enjoyed to eat and what thrived in their environment. Dandelion is a bit of a master of being able to grow in many places and environments so it was a good choice from that perspective, plus dandelion is delicious and so many parts are used for food and medicine. The leaves, the flowers and roots are all used in various ways (please see the entry on dandelion later in the book). The concept of cultivating a plant that we in our modern world call a weed is a strange and foreign one because we now have the luxury of easy access to food on a daily basis.

Our food supply and farming systems are very much driven by profit and demand, not by nutrition and taste. As a herbalist it pains me seeing folk eating a well-balanced diet but not getting full nutrition from it; as a forager it pains me to see the bland offerings in our modern vegetables and food. We deserve to enjoy the full taste of our food. There are folk who have never tasted the real taste of, say, a tomato picked straight from the bush or a carrot straight out of the ground. But this sad state of affairs is changing as we look towards local and sustainable methods for food production and supply. Be warned, though: once you taste real food and its fuller flavour you will find it hard to go back to blander mass-produced items. Adding some foraged foods to your diet will really add flavour and nutrition to your plate.

Our ancestors had to eat what was around them and what could grow in their environment. We have almost a global larder now. This comes at a price, though, as the amount of transportation required means the produce is not at its best in terms of ripeness and therefore flavour and nutrition. Then add in the environmental cost of shipping our food to our plates. The benefits of choosing local, sustainable and fresher food far outweigh eating the far-flung, exotic but poor nutritional offerings from other places.

So I would like to look at what food we can prepare for ourselves in our kitchens that will excite our taste buds and provide more nutrition for us. In times gone by folk used to preserve a lot of the harvest through various methods that we don't employ in the same way anymore. We have freezers and fridges that prolong the shelf life of our food. The very act of gathering your food and preserving will feel very wholesome and bring you closer to nature. I would like to guide you on how to do this.

Seasons and senses
Phenology is the study of seasonality. It combines ecology with meteorology. Our ancestors did not know this word but they understood it at a deeper level than anyone studying it! In a traditional farming calendar folk knew when the shortest and longest day were as it dictated the length of time that work could be done and the temperature. Weather plays a huge role in how crops develop and therefore on yields. This hasn't changed much: we still see crops failing from a diversion of normal weather patterns for that year.

Foraging

A few years ago the wheat crop didn't produce the same yield, and the price went up for flour and all wheat products. This would have been similar in years gone by but the difference is that it was not money that was the base line and more whether there was enough of that crop to take folk through the rest of the year in the community relying on it. This can work the other way in that there can be bumper harvests some years, and then the need to preserve that crop becomes the issue.

Barley in Scotland is an interesting case in that years ago if there was an abundance of barley it ended up being distilled and turned into an alcoholic beverage. It was a great way to preserve the harvest. This was the beginnings of whisky. Some years there are bigger harvests than others, and this varies from plant to plant. On the years there is an abundance we preserve the

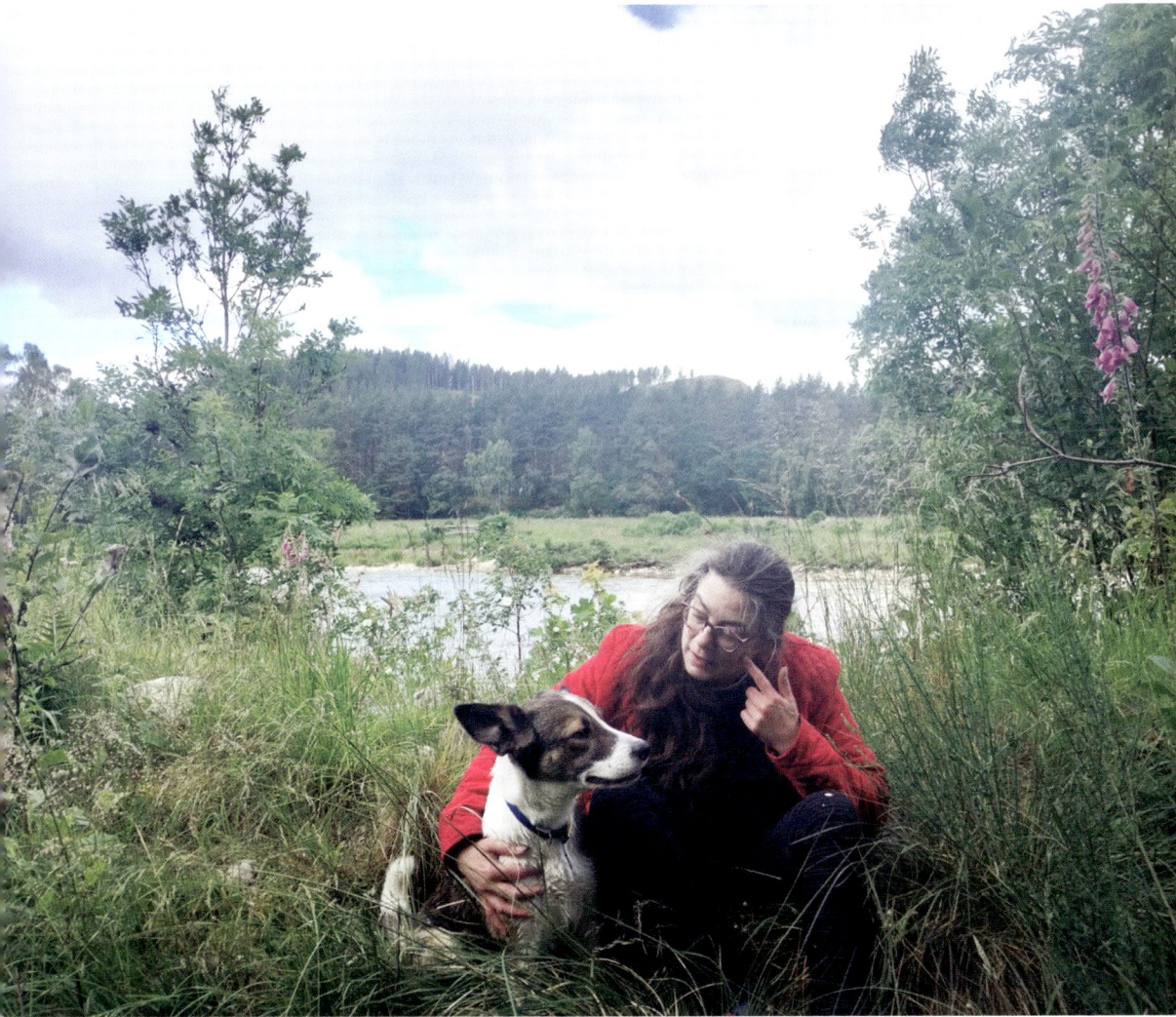

harvest in various ways, such as pickles, ferments and chutneys, to take us into Winter and hopefully through to the next harvest. Please see the recipes section below.

We use our senses constantly and automatically. We look where we are going, we listen for sounds like a timer, a notification on our phones or alarm clock, perhaps the sound of traffic so we don't get run over. We also listen to the sounds of birds, wind, rain. Even the sound of snow, which magically dampens sound but also creates its own sound when walking on it or made it into snowballs. They are very different sounds that evoke different feelings and thoughts.

When we are learning about a plant, where it is located and what it looks like, we also learn about its smell, taste and even the sounds it makes. Take broom on a warm sunny day, when the seed pods release their seeds with an audible pop. It's a fantastic sound and one that reminds me of bright sunshiny days. I'm currently writing this in –5C in February, albeit indoors with the heating on. So it's a lovely memory to evoke, remember and look forward to.

Using your senses to learn good identification skills is essential. You use most of them without even thinking. I wonder if our ancestors had other senses that they possibly used. Some studies suggest we have more than five senses. One even suggests we have 21 senses. This is not beyond the realms of belief as birds use electromagnetic fields to find their way. I wonder if they know they are doing this or is it something we have observed.

For me intuition is one of those 'senses' or perceptions. For some this seems almost mystical, but I think another level of sensory awareness is something we all have. It is often not recognised by folk as they don't know it exists, are not aware of it or if they do know find it hard to recognise. I do feel some of our senses are drowned out by modern life and the stresses this can bring. We can so busy there isn't enough time to relax, and with so many modern digital devices demanding our attention it is hard to listen to ourselves.

In one of Ellis Peters's novels the monk Brother Cadfael says: 'Sometimes I think the senses are the gateway to the soul and we should celebrate them more.' How would you do this? Smell a fragrant flower, eat a delicious meal, stand in the woods or forest and enjoy the surroundings and feeling? The sounds of a river and bird song?

Foraging

Connection and relationship

Connection. What does it mean? How do we know it? Do we see it, hear it or feel it? The simple answer is all of them, and probably some we haven't put a name to yet.

We feel connection in my places and with many folk. We feel it just saying hello to someone in the street, or even without speech we can convey our feelings with a smile. It is a simple act that says deep down all is okay and there is no threat here. We feel it in the woods, on a beach, beside a river and up a mountain looking at the scenery. We feel it at a concert/gig/festival with the music and then with the camaraderie of sharing that experience with the crowd.

The joy of getting closer to nature through foraging and being out in nature can't be described well by words. Words feel ill equipped to convey the feeling that is connection. The best way to know the feeling is to go and be shown or feel it for yourself. We get a sense of it when we hear birds singing and

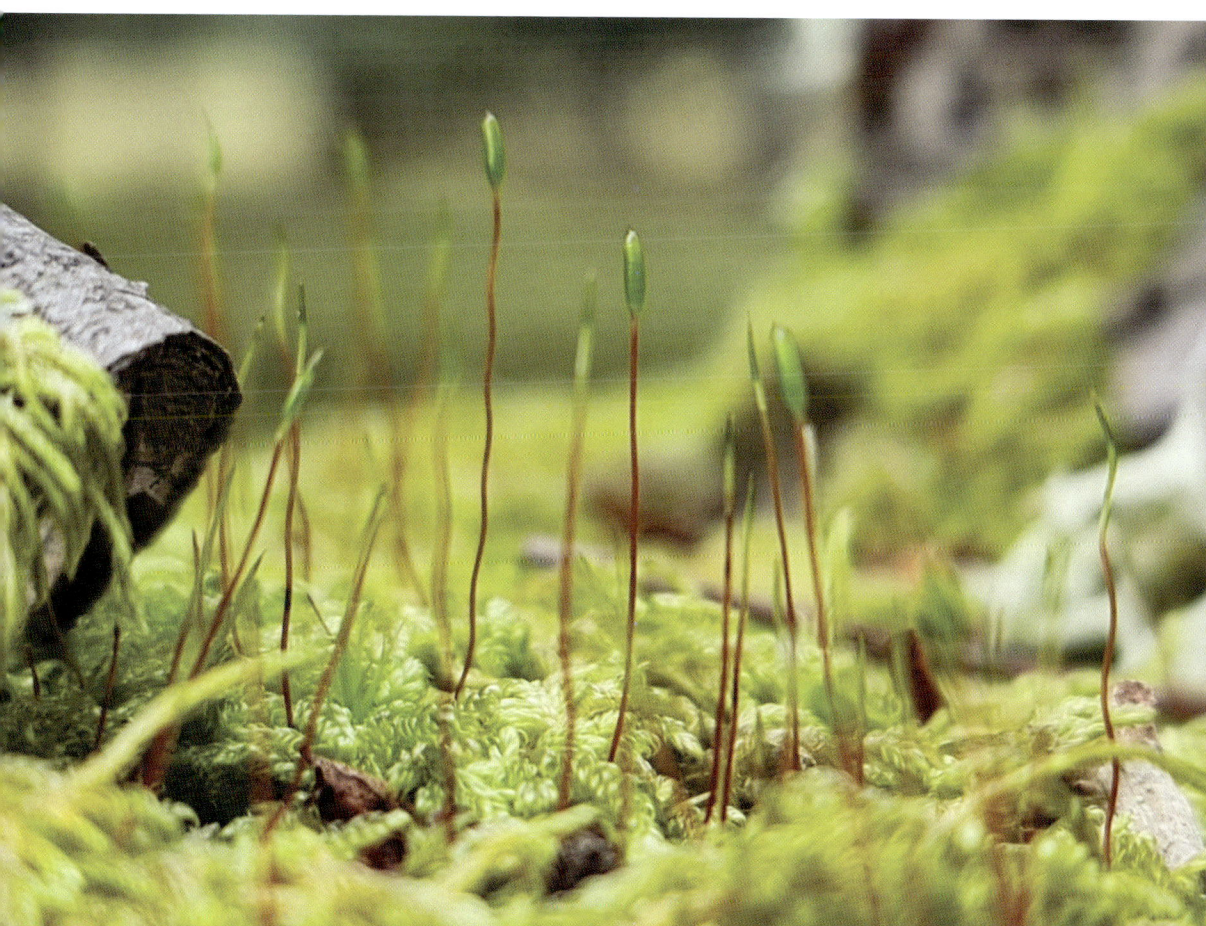

when we look out to sea. It's also being part of the silence and calmness. We all know that our modern culture runs too fast and that this causes us a level of stress that is unsustainable long term; we also know it can be countered by deepening your connection with nature.

The time, energy and effort required of any relationship is the same for our relationship and connection with nature. If you don't make the effort to relax and use your senses in nature you won't appreciate it in the same way. If you brisk-walk along the river you will miss some aspects of your surroundings. Learn to take a slower mindset into nature.

Yes, there are times when having to walk your dog before work where your mind won't have time to relax as you are getting ready for the day ahead. The more time you spend in nature the quicker the connection and feeling arises. So when you do have to do that speedier walk owing to time and day-to-day commitments after experiencing more connected walks you will find you connect quicker on those walks. Simply get outside more and slow down.

Often on a walk I gain a lot more than I give, and the interactions with nature feel different and more open. It is a privilege to be able to see that happen to people on a walk or workshop when they learn more of the detail of plants and fungi.

The idea of connection and the reality can be different depending on our expectations. For example, you might want to go out and be immersed in nature while wanting to hear birds sing. You go out into the woods, don't hear many birds but instead see some amazing lichen that fascinates you. The ability to be open to hear the bird song allowed you to slow down and refocus. This then let you see the detail of the lichen and be absorbed by it for a while. Science is a very useful tool for understanding so much of our world and in good detail. I use science all the time, looking for recent studies that explain a bit more about a plant or fungi, often confirming what we already used traditionally and sometimes leading us off into different areas. I thank science for seeing the world in a different way, and it has a place in our understanding of nature.

I studied mathematics with the Open University years ago, choosing it because it was a subject I was good at in school, contrary to a lot of people's experience with it. I found the patterns that formed with maths interesting and developed a love for fractals. When I discovered that nature produced fractals all the time I was amazed. Nature and maths, which are often seen as opposite subjects, have a deep common thread.

Identify your plants properly!
Plant identification is very important and should never be overlooked if you take up foraging. Getting it wrong can have serious consequences. Note that this book is not about identification because there are already plenty of very good books out there to help you with botany and detailed plant ID. The best way to learn is to go out with someone who already has those skills. And please do not get over-confident and forget the basics. Always check!

Here's a personal example. A few years ago I took a delightful lady, Michelle Chan, on a walk. She really is a 'breath of fresh air' woman and we chatted all the way round about various subjects. I enjoyed her company immensely. We looked at and tasted numerous plants, and as we were coming to the end of the walk, I stopped and picked a seed, thinking it was a common hogweed seed. There had been one in that location the year before, so I didn't check.
As we gently nibbled the seed we agreed it didn't have any flavour. Common hogweed seeds have a strong flavour that can take a short while to develop. But nothing happened with this seed. I then checked the plant … it wasn't common hogweed! What was it? It wasn't poison hemlock or hemlock water dropwort, poisonous species in the same family.

My mind started to whir and I thought 'damn, that looks like cowbane'. Cowbane can also kill you but you need to consume 5% of your body weight for ill effects to happen, and these effects take 15 minutes to an hour to show. The effect is similar to the poisoning from hemlock where the nervous system starts to shut down from the peripheral to the central, hence starting at the hands and feet and finishing with your core nervous system. This would eventually lead to the lungs and heart not working and therefore death.

As we finished our walk I took solace in the fact we had only nibbled the seed and not eaten more of it, but of course I was worried. We had another hour together after the walk with a wild cocktail masterclass from the excellent mixologist Marco Fante. I had worked with Marco creating cocktails for Elsa's Bar so I mentioned to him we had potentially nibbled a cowbane. So he understood why we were occasionally checking that the sensation was still in our feet and hands while in his class. The atmosphere was all very light-hearted and relaxed.

I knew that if it was cowbane we had consumed we hadn't swallowed enough for serious effects. Afterwards I checked the full identification of the plant, and it turned out to be a lesser-leaved hogweed, a plant whose seeds you can nibble safely. If I had simply checked the plant while I was picking all of that worry would not have happened.

I messaged Michelle as soon as I had identified the plant so that she didn't worry. She thanked me and in the morning sent me an email to say she was alive! It was said tongue in cheek, but nonetheless it was a situation that could have been avoided if I had followed the correct procedure and not been over-confident or blasé about identification that day. So please learn from my lesson and always, always identify to 100% before picking and eating. I have not made that mistake again and always check now.

Information in the community
Scotland's traditional medicine was passed on orally rather than being written down. A fair amount of smaller cultures continue with oral traditions as their method to pass on information. This keeps it within the community and not into the wider world. In our modern world there is so much information it can be dizzying. A lot of it is wrong information, and sometimes downright lies trying to be put across as truth.

The idea of keeping information in a community means it is less likely to be incorrectly passed on. Learning is best done by being shown by someone who knows what they are doing. I feel this rings true of foraging and herbal medicine. I've been lucky enough to have been taught both by some of the best minds and souls in Scotland and beyond. Some of these you would not know the names of let alone meet them on social media as they choose to be quietly doing their work and not in the limelight. I urge you to seek out folk who truly know what they are doing and learn from them directly. This is where culture and community are important. This is a world away from commercialism, ego and status. Songs and stories carried meanings and information.

The forager's calendar
We are aware of the seasons mostly because of the weather. For most people in the past they would have been more aware of the changes in the seasons for growing crops, foraging, hunting. Lacking modern lighting made daylight more important for what folk could do and not do. The four seasons we have in Scotland are sometimes represented as life and death and renewal. Spring is the beginning of life and Winter as the death when a lot of the plants put their energy into their roots and lay dormant for a few months.

The significant days are important as they mark the seasons and the changes in the weather. That is their main purpose: to collectively mark the change. Everyone knew when it was in times before newspapers and the internet. There have been many days added to our calendar year to celebrate other aspects of our modern culture. The days listed below are in relation to the northern hemisphere and the seasons experienced.

- Summer Solstice – longest day and shortest night.
- Winter Solstice – shortest day and longest night.
- Spring Equinox – equal day and night.
- Autumn Equinox – equal day and night.

Plants and their medicinal and ethnobotanical uses, for example, for thatching, dyeing and so on, have shaped Scotland's progress and into the modern world. In the days before travel and trade, what was around you was your larder and medicine cabinet. One example of how the plants were important is the attributing of plants and trees to the Gaelic alphabet. It shows folks' connection to them.

Plants and the alphabet

I'm using the Ogham as laid out by Mary Beith in her excellent book *A'chraobh: The Tree* (2000).

B – birch – *beithe*
L – rowan – *caorann*
N – ash – *uinnseann*
F – alder – *fearn*
S – willow – *seileach* or *sail*
H – hawthorn – s*githeach* or *droigheann*
D – oak – *darach*
T – holly – *cuileann*
C – hazel – *calltainn*
M – vine – *crann-fiona*
G – ivy – *eidheann* or *iadhslat*
P – peith – *peith* [viburnum]
R – elder – *ruis*
A – wych elm – *leamhan*
O – gorse – *conasg*
U – heather – *fraoch*
E – aspen – *eadha*
I – yew – *iubhar*

Old stories set in nature

As with a lot of languages in more remote and rural areas the language is shaped significantly around nature. In the same way the Inuit have many names for snow, Gaelic has several names for water: the water from the sky called rain is different from the water out of our taps and the water in the burn. One name that we are more familiar with is one of Scotland's leading exports, whisky – *uisge beatha* – water of life.

Life is stories. We have always loved stories from being a child to an adult. In years gone by and sometimes now there are stories that give us life advice or pinpoint information for us – like saying where an abundant patch of nettles is and their uses. In the modern world stories have become so numerous, and of course not all of them are true. As a society we turned more to stories and nature in the lockdowns, and we found comfort in regrounding ourselves away a bit from the reality of what is happening around us. Escapism, but finding grounding in old stories often set in nature.

Our connection with nature and the land is often seen in names – how we named the rivers, mountains, hills, lochs and places. Names are interesting, and in themselves words that give identity and can mark a time in history. This weekend I was reminded of the way that place names are created and at times changed owing to events that happen in a particular place. There are lots of stories of events that happened in places, for example, where two lovers had hung out away from society for a while; usually a tragic event happened and one or both of them lost their lives where they were hiding, and the crag where they were hiding is named after them. Scotland is littered with these renamings after events, thankfully not all of them tragic.

Before the days of Google Maps and even paper maps we would have places in the landscape that folk would meet at. These were called Clachan stones. Quite simply, these would be obvious stones in the landscape that everyone in the local community would know.

There is connection of place to ancient spirits and ancestors, with otherworldly and marked days of the year. This requires more than just being in nature, this requires *feeling* nature. It joins the living and the dead, the past and the present. It offers a deeper sense of belonging and a binding to culture.

Plants

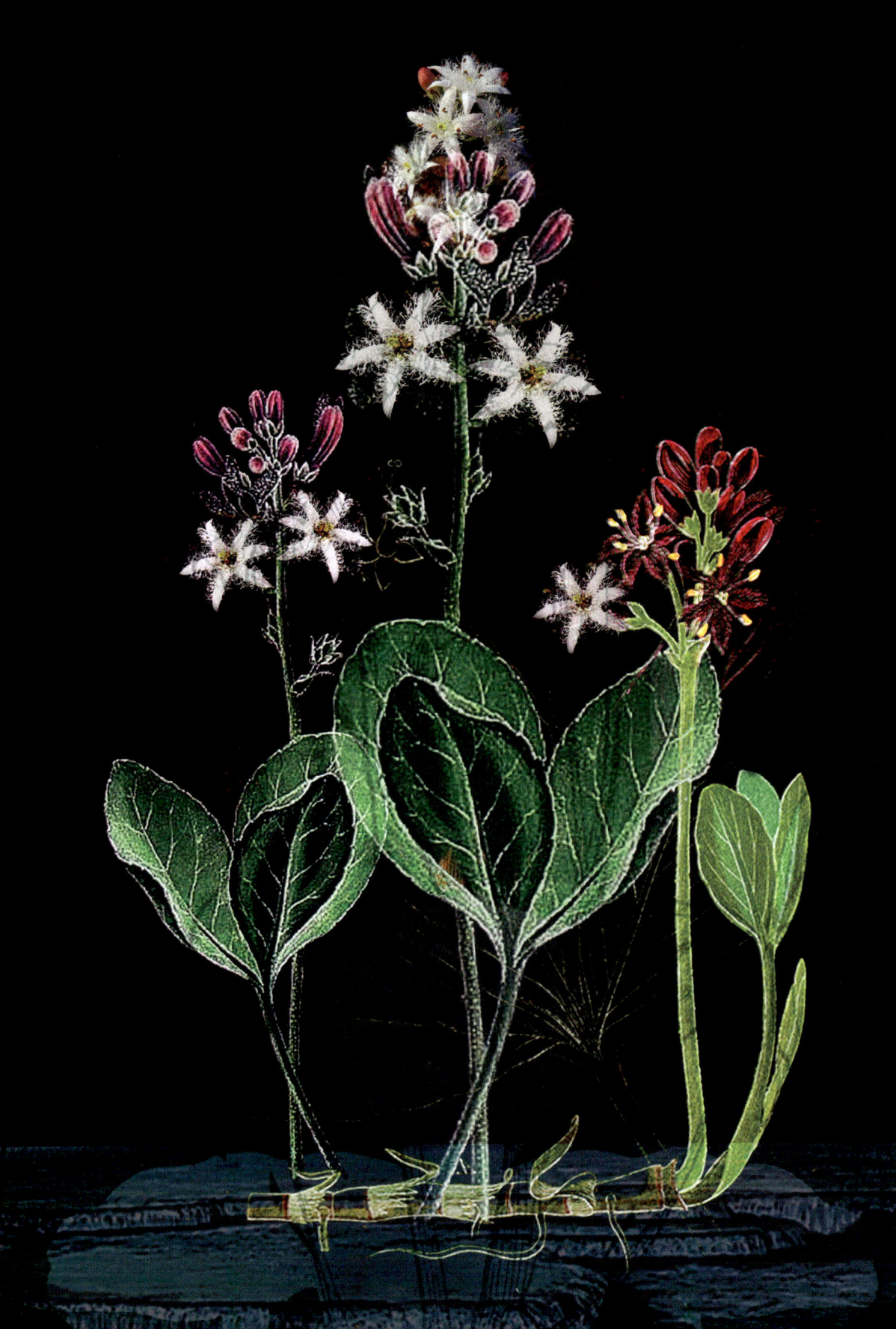

Bogbean

Menyanthes trifoliata

Gaelic names: Trì-bhileach; Lus nan Laogh

Menyanthaceae

Parts used – leaves

I was first introduced to bogbean by excellent neighbours on the Isle of Lewis, John M. and Margaret MacLeod. I have very fond memories of spending time with them learning Gaelic and occasionally going fishing together.

Margaret broke her wrist on the road one day – the wrist has many small bones in it, and Margaret had done a grand job of breaking many of them. While she was recovering John looked after her. She was much more static than usual, and a leg ulcer started to appear on the lower part of one of her legs.

So John went out and collected bogbean leaves from the local lochan (small loch). He simmered them for eight hours, and then Margaret drank shot-sized amounts on a daily basis – with it being Lewis measures, this was about 50ml each day. She did this for a month and the leg ulcer started to clear up. The local doctor was amazed.

Bogbean is a very bitter plant, and when John offered a glass to me he said, 'if you can drink whisky you can drink this'. He knew I could drink whisky as we had many a dram together, and I can still see the glint in his eye as I took it. It was indeed bitter, and I must have pulled a face, as John smiled.

John M. and many others knew bogbean as a blood purifier and a plant that helps cleanse the liver. It is a bitter herb useful for all sorts of stomach pains, particularly those caused by ulcers.

The German name is *Scharbock*, a corruption of the old Latin word *scorbutus*, which was the name for scurvy, and it was used for this condition.

It has been used for sluggish digestion. With chronic diseases, particularly arthritis and digestive issues, the routes of elimination get sluggish and toxins can build up, making the condition worse.

It contains coumarins, including scopoletin, scoparone and bryalin. These have shown choleretic and cholagogue qualities and are anti-hepatotoxic.

The iridiod glycosides in bogbean – dihydromenthiafolin, menthyafolin, menyanthin, sweroside and loganin – have aperient and laxative activity, and are enhanced by the phenolic acids present.

Its secoiridoids are very bitter and stimulate the taste buds, which increases gastric secretions and therefore improves appetite.

Bogbean also contains betulinic acid, tannins, pyridine alkaloids – gentainine, gentainadine and inulin – and the root has quantities of quercetin, rutin, salicylic acid and saponins.

It has antibacterial properties based on its vitamin C and gentianin content. Other uses for it include to treat rheumatism, skin diseases and liver issues.

In the Western Isles it was a highly valued plant, especially in tonic form. Barbara Fairweather gives a recipe from Glencoe, where within living memory a bogbean paste was made in a stone jar and simmered on an old range for a few hours. It was diluted and drunk as a spring tonic.

It also went into a homemade beer until being replaced by hops. The beer would be stored away until required.

In her book *Healing Threads* Mary Beith recommends taking a teaspoon a day for a persistent cough. The juice was given for TB. A bogbean poultice was made for boils and skin eruptions. Pain in the side resulting from jaundice was once treated using wild raspberry, wild mint and bogbean.

In the Uists bogbean was used for constipation. John Lightfoot in 1777 recommended it as a tea to help strengthen a weak stomach.

Henri Leclerc, the founder of phytotherapy, said bogbean is useful and effective for headaches associated with atonic dyspepsia.

It has a beautiful white, feathery flower.

Cautions
Large doses of bogbean are emetic. Not to be used for diarrhoea or with colitis.

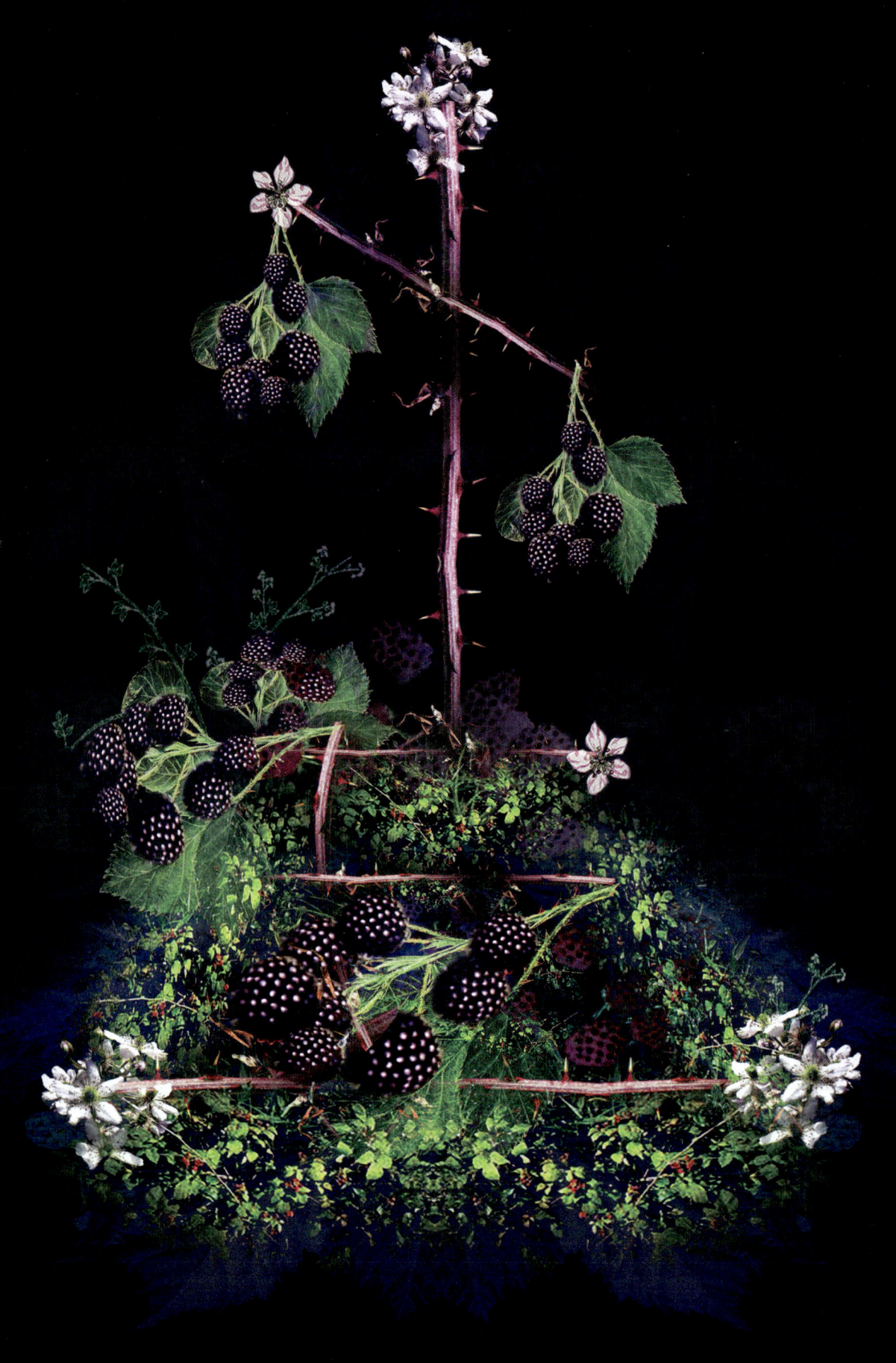

Bramble

Rubus fruticosus

Gaelic name: Dris

Rosaceae

Parts used – leaves and fruit

As mentioned before, bramble was my first foraged plant when a child. I had discovered nettle and dandelion when weeding, and then diligently read about them in Mrs Grieve's *A Modern Herbal*. But for going out and gathering plants it was bramble that I was taught about, and I enjoyed all the resulting pies and crumbles at home. My Mum said we were not to take the fruit in October. She had had this wisdom passed on to her. I enquired why. My Mum said because in October brambles become the devil's own. I didn't accept this as an answer and soon learnt it was actually because on aging they become tasteless, mouldy and maggot-infested.

In 1777 John Lightfoot wrote that bramble root and pennyroyal were given for bronchitis and asthma. Erysipelas was treated with a poultice of the leaves. The Greeks recorded that an unspecified part of bramble was used for gout.

Francis Buchanan wrote in *The Scottish Naturalist* in 1876 that the berries were often eaten and afforded a good jelly.

Sore throats were treated with the fruit as they contain a fair amount of vitamin C. This remedy is still used today for sore throats and mouths.

The berries also contain potassium, magnesium, calcium, omega 3 and 6, vitamin A, the Bs, C, E and K.

All dark fruits contain anthocyanins. Bramble leaves contain tannins, which supports their traditional use for treating diarrhoea.

Margaret Bennett, Martyn Bennett's Mum, said a bramble branch used to be placed above a door to ward off evil. The Gaelic name is directly translated as 'blessed bramble'.

Christ was said to have used a bramble switch to drive his donkey as he rode to Jerusalem before expelling the money lenders from the temple.

In 2006, a Forestry Commission research paper by Marla Emery and colleagues, *Wild Harvests from Scottish Woodlands*, showed that almost a quarter of people in Scotland had picked brambles in the previous five years.

Cautions

None known.

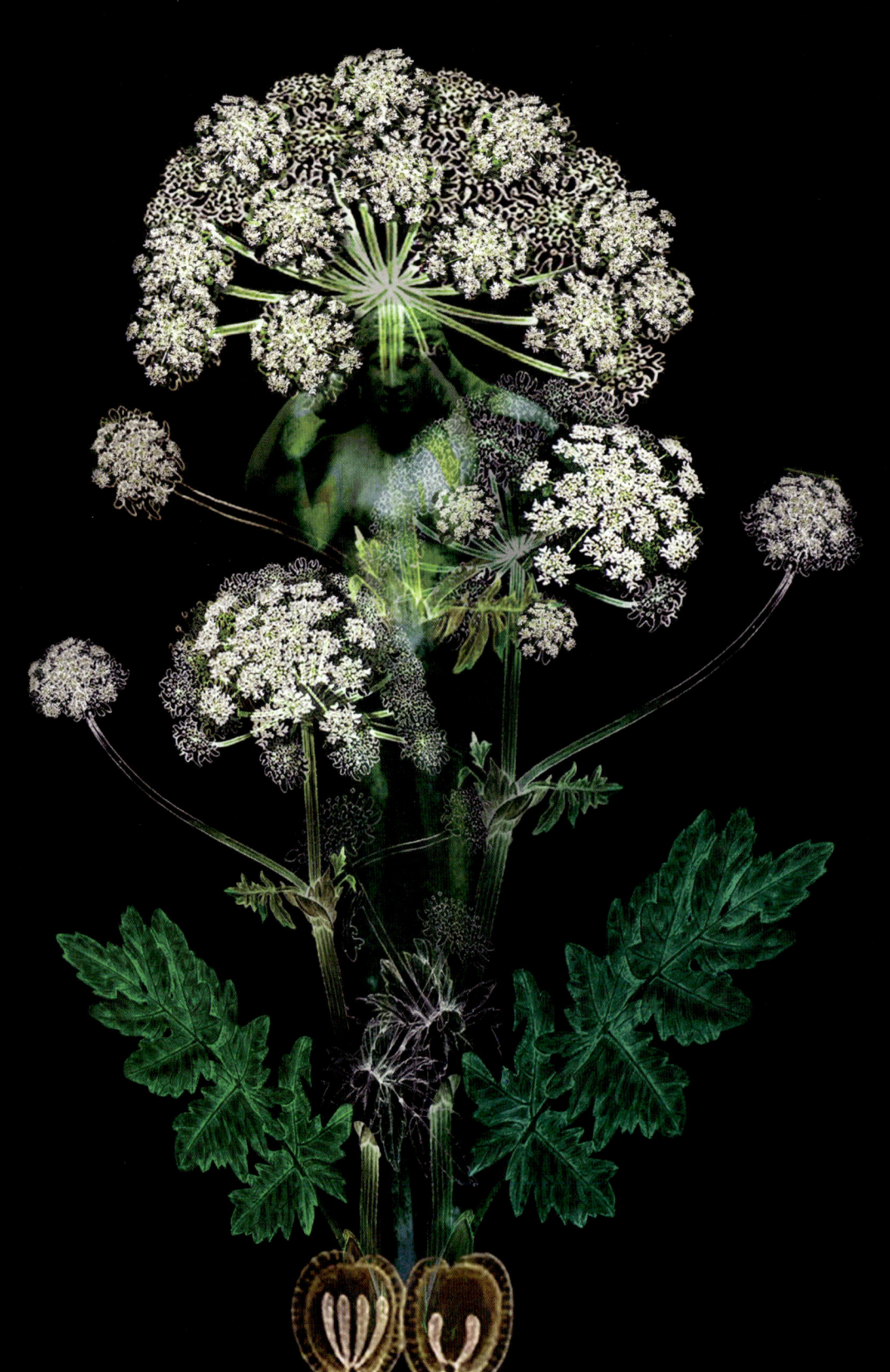

Common hogweed

Heracleum sphondylium

Gaelic name: Odharan

Apiaceae

Parts used – young leaf, flower buds, young shoots, seeds

This is a strong, upright plant, reflected in its Latin name *Heracleum*, meaning pertaining to Hercules. The common name hogweed is from it being used as a pig food.

Common hogweed often gets mistakenly mixed up with giant hogweed. These two related plants are significantly different in size once you have seen them – giant hogweed is very tall, up to 4m high, and is easily seen in its environment, along water courses and rivers.

Common hogweed, on the other hand, is much smaller, at about half the height, and is often found along roadsides and walkways. As you drive past it can be seen as one of the abundant wild white flowers of June and July.

On closer examination when you walk by you will see the large, divided leaf of common hogweed is different from the other umbelliferous white flowers you may see in summer, which will often be cow parsley.

Common hogweed's flower has a musty smell found enjoyable by some and repellent to others. Either way for you, lots of insects love this plant – over a hundred species of insects visit.

Common hogweed contains furanocoumarins, which can cause skin reactions such as blistering and a burning reaction. This is much more likely to happen in sunlight, so the advice is pick the young shoots on a dull day. These young shoots are tasty pan-fried with butter and garlic. The flowerheads have similarities to courgette flowers, and can be cooked and used in the same way as them.

The seeds have an interesting flavour that remind me of oranges and cardamom as well as a unique strong flavour of their own. The immature green and ripe beige-coloured seeds have their own distinct flavours.

As collectors and foragers, in order to feel safe and familiar we look for flavours in the wild that are similar to those we already know. We find that nettles taste like spinach. There are plenty of flavours in the wild that are new and unfamiliar to us, and the flavour of hogweed seeds is where I started to really notice that.

I recently did a talk about foraging in Ballater for a local group. As I was talking about common hogweed and the blistering it can cause, one gentlemen piped up and said, 'Oh, that's what caused the marks we had on our lips when we used them as blowpipes as a child.' That made a fair number of folk smile, and you could almost visibly see a wave of realisation spread through the room.

My first introduction to this plant was through Mark Williams of Galloway Wild Foods on a foraging day he did for herbalists. We had such fun and learnt loads – thanks, Mark.

Scientific research shows even more interesting results, and we are in the early stages of understanding this plant a bit more.

The only known medicinal use for me is one that is pretty much across the board for the Apaciae (formerly the Umbelliferae) family, namely as a digestive that aids digestion and helps it run a bit smoother. I haven't used common hogweed as a medicine, but looking into it has been very interesting. For example, the extracted stem juice was applied to warts and the pollen was dusted onto sores. Looking further back:

- In the 16th century John Gerard used it for headaches and lethargy.
- In the 17th century it was mentioned by Nicholas Culpeper for treating epilepsy and jaundice.
- In the 18th century on Mull it was used as a digestive.

– Also in the 18th century Carl Linnaeus used hogweed as a sedative.

A fermented soup is made of hogweed leaves in Poland and Lithuania.

In 1548, the herbalist William Turner was first to call it cow parsnip. In North America cow parsnip was one of the most used Native American wild foods. It is recorded to be the same for pre-revolutionary Russia and the Baltic states as a widely used food.
Medicinally, in North America the root was used in teas and tinctures for colic, cramps, headaches, colds, flu and TB, while also applied externally for sores, bruises, stiff joints and active boils.

In modern France it is has been recorded as an aphrodisiac and for high blood pressure. In Sweden and East Germany it is used as a sedative.

In Europe generally it was used as an amphoteric for the nervous system, meaning that it acted as both a stimulant and as a sedative,. This sounds contradictory but is in fact how the plant works in normalising bodily function.

The late William LeSassier's work, cited by Matthew Wood, established that chewing common hogweed seeds heightens sensitivity and confers psychic benefits.

In 21st-century research, common hogweed has been shown to have the following actions:

2006 antifungal, anti mycobacterial and antiviral.
2008 anti-asthmatic, memory effects, including improving alertness.
2010 antimycobacterial elements identified, including several furanocourmarins – supports the traditional use for treating infectious diseases, including TB.
2013 vasorelaxant properties found, supporting treatment for high blood pressure.
2014 the essential oil showed the compound octyl butyrate, which is cytotoxic to certain melanoma and carcinoma cells.

This all indicates an exciting start to looking at the science for this plant.

Cautions

Some folk get a contact dermatitis from touching the plant and some from the sap, which worsens in sunlight. Please be careful handling this plant, and obviously don't eat it if you get a reaction.

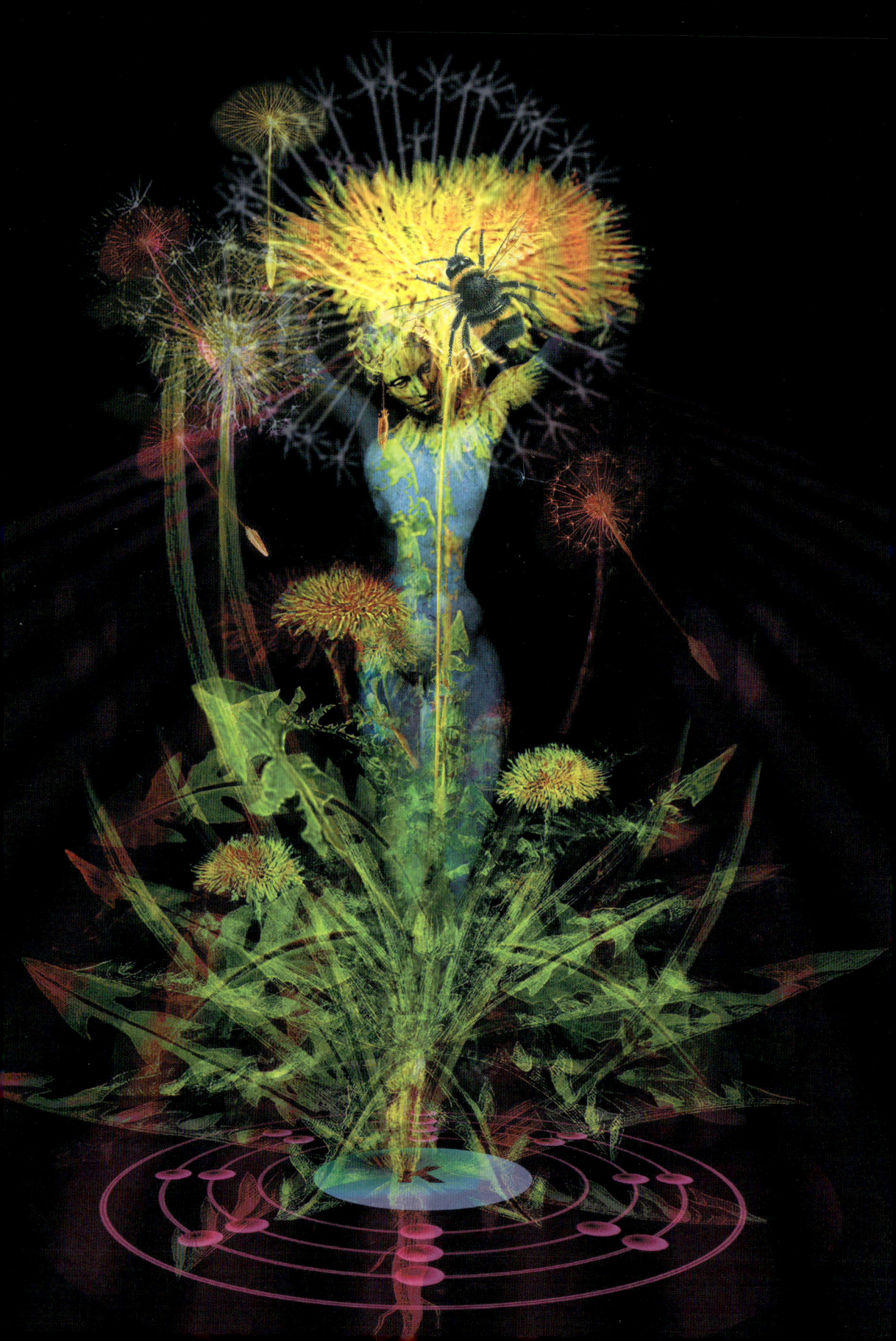

Dandelion

Taraxacum officinale

Gaelic name: Beàrnan Brìghde

Asteraceae

Parts used – leaf, root and flower

A very familiar plant to many people. Its bright yellow and showy flowers are a welcome sight in April.

One of its common names, *Piss en lit*, indicates dandelion's diuretic uses, and the name *Dent de lion* is thought to be a symbol of the lion, meaning the sun. Dandelion only shows its flowers in sunlight, not on a dull day, which indicates how it got this name, but the lion's teeth appearance of some of the leaves could also be another source. Its Chinese name translates as yellow-flowered earth nail, which I'm sure many a gardener will resonate with.

During the lockdowns I was writing a nature newsletter for The Fife Arms in Braemar. I decided to write about dandelion and did some research. One thing I discovered was that the settlers to America had taken dandelion with them intentionally to grow for food and medicine. When more affluence occurred the people were able to turn their growing patches into lawn areas and lawns became a symbol of status. I'm very aware that these days we spend time weeding dandelion from our lawns.

The leaf is a frequent addition to salads in Europe, adding a sweet bitterness that is delicious. It is a mild diuretic, as we have seen, and also has high levels of potassium in the leaf, which can help us keep a good mineral balance in the body.

The flowers can be used to make wine, fritters and a flower-based honey – great if you are vegan or choose not to use bee products. The honey does use a lot of sugar, though, and really ends up tasting like honey.

The roasted root was used as a coffee substitute in years gone by. This does not contain caffeine, though. It does have a distinctive coffee flavour, but when I make a syrup of it has chocolate and caramel in there too. And it makes a great white Russian cocktail.

The root also contains inulin, which is a prebiotic to probiotics and helps improve gut flora and the microbiome.

It also contains bitter glycosides, phytosterols, tannins, vitamins A, B and C, zinc and manganese. The pollen is antimicrobial and has been shown to be useful against *Proteus mirabilis*, *Escherichia coli* and species of *Salmonella*.

Dandelion leaf and root have been used effectively in herbal medicine for a long time. The leaf is also a mild heptalogue, which means it gently moves bile through the liver. The root has a stronger effect on the liver and therefore the digestive system.

There has been some interesting research on the root in the last few years, including at Windsor University, which has been conducting a human trial for leukaemia, pancreatic and colon cancers.

Modern research papers have shown it to have an effect similar to the diuretic frusemide.

It was mentioned in Chinese medicine in AD 659 and in European medicine around 1485. Arabs physicians used it in the 11th century, and it became an official drug by the 16th century. The Physicians of Myddfai in Wales (from the 13th century) mention it in their literature. And Nicholas Culpeper wrote in 1652: 'By the bitterness [it] doth more open and cleanse and is therefore very effectual for the obstructions of the liver, gall and spleen and the diseases that arise from them, as the jaundice.'

In Glencoe dandelion leaves between bread and butter were eaten as an old cure for stomach ulcers.

The white sap of the stalks of dandelion changes your skin colour temporarily, and you can create designs and patterns with this sap. It was also used to remove warts.

When I was a kid we would use dandelion seedheads to see if somebody loved us or not. We would blow into the seedhead, say he loves me and then with the next blow say he loves me not. The last blow that cleared the seedhead of all seeds was your answer.

Cautions

None known.

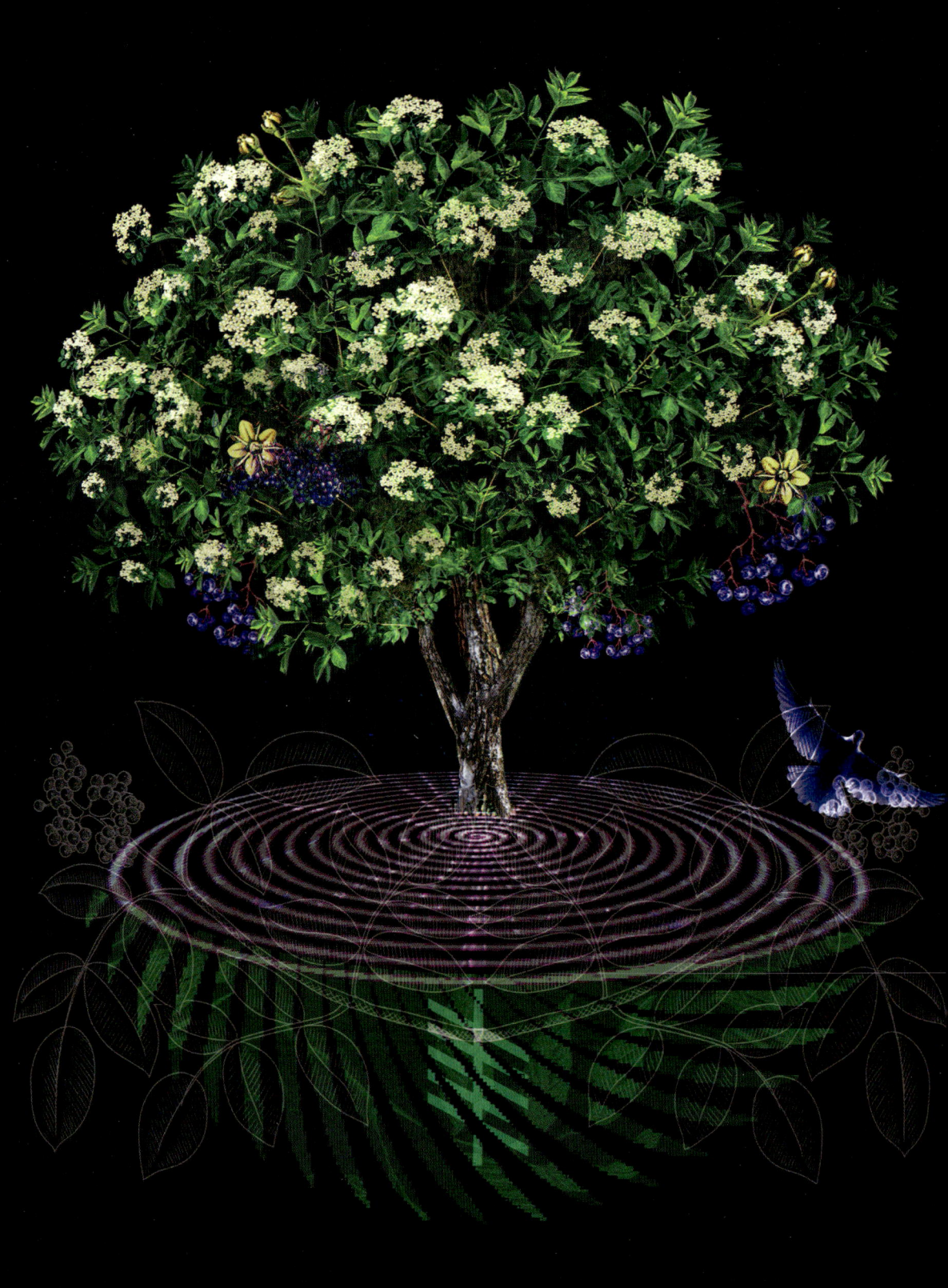

Elderberry

Sambucus nigra

Gaelic name: Droman; Ruis

Adoxaceae

Parts used – flower and fruit

These days when folk think of elder they often think of the flowers, and the berries tend to be forgotten about. This is a flavour and medicinal oversight. The robust and deep flavour of the berries is wonderful.

It is important not to use any of the stalks in elder recipes as they contain small amounts of cyanide.

The flowers contain volatile oils, flavonoids including rutin, vitamins A and C, tannins, mucilage and sterols.

Elder is a diaphoretic, a warming expectorant, anticatarrhal, anti-inflammatory and diuretic. The berries are laxative and antiviral.

European history is littered with reverence for elder. Hippocrates (c. 460 BC to c.370 BC) mentioned it. It is a traditional and old herbal tea for colds. John Evelyn's *Sylva* of 1664 said: 'If the medicinal properties of the leaves, bark, berries &c. were thoroughly known, I cannot tell what our country-men could ail, for which he might not fetch a remedy from every hedge, either for sickness or wound.'

In 1777 John Lightfoot related that the inner bark matured in white wine was a gentle carthartic and deobstructrent that would get bodily fluids moving again. The bruised leaves were used in combating pleurisy and the juice of the dried berries as an aid against indigestion.

A much-believed superstition was that elder was the tree that Judas hung himself on, which was also why it smelled so bad at Easter time.

It is also a sacred tree, a tree of the Ogham that was not to be cut down. It was held in such reverence that folk in the Highlands and Islands would have a nod to the elder tree as they walked past.

The pollen was important, and the tree was planted to protect to keep witches at bay. The sap was said to activate the second sight in those who had it.

There were two dates, at summer solstice and all hallow's eve, in which standing or sleeping under an elder tree on a fairy hill would allow a seer to see fairies.

Cautions
The raw berries are emetic. The leaf and stem are mildly toxic. It is important not to use any of the stalks in elder recipes as they contain small amounts of cyanide.

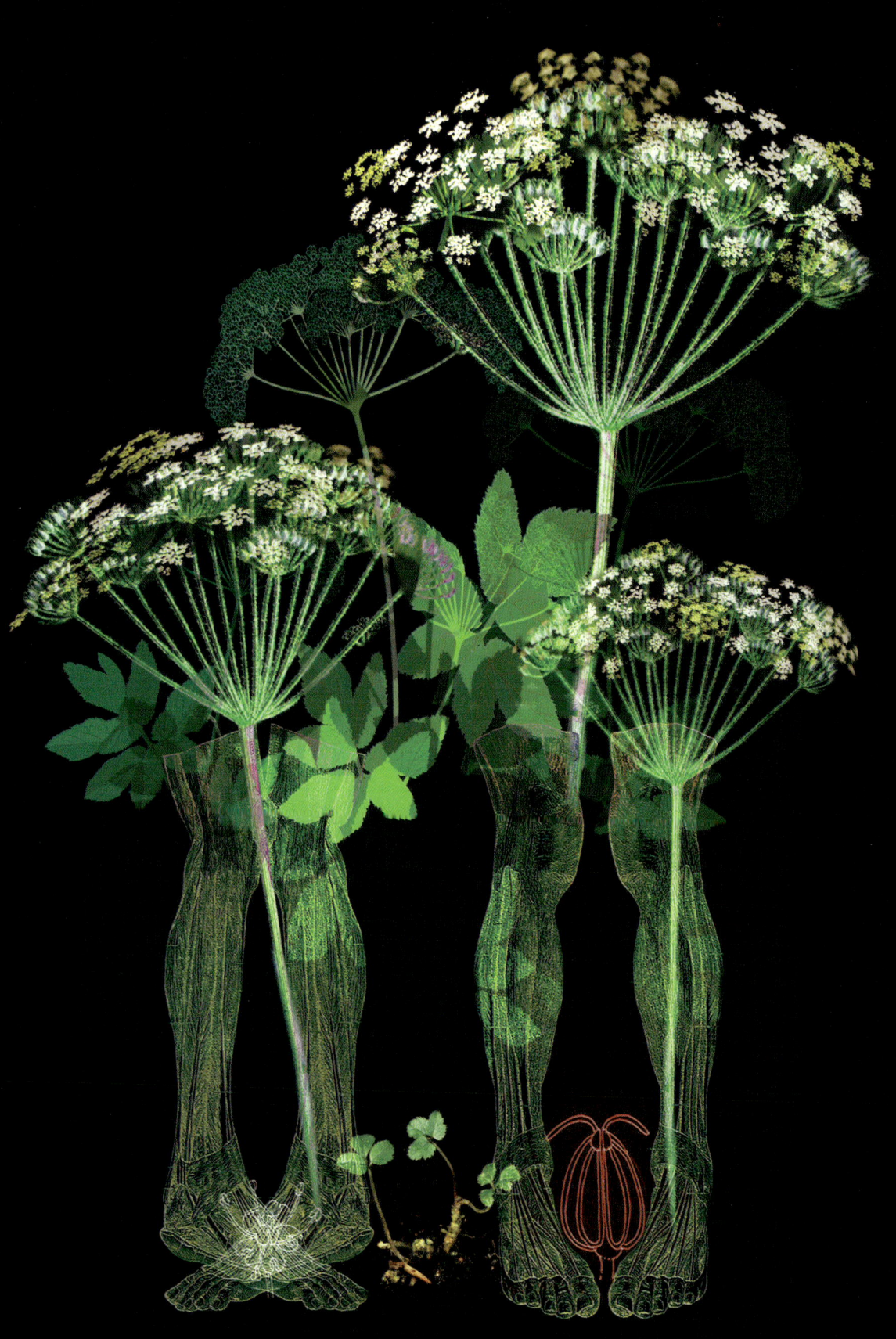

Ground elder

Aegopodium podagraria

Gaelic name: Lus an Easbaig

Apiaceae

Parts used – young leaf

Ground elder is also known as goutweed and bishops weed.

It appears early in the year, from late March onwards. It is always the young waxy-looking shiny leaves that are the best to eat. They taste of parsley and celery at the same time – delicious.

Ground elder is thought to have been brought to Britain by the Romans as a source of food and medicine. The common name goutweed reflects its ability to help pull impurities from the joints and therefore help with gout and arthritis. Its other name, bishops weed, is either from the clergy's drinking habits and their resulting gout or because the plant grew in monastic gardens.

Saint Gerard of Toul (935–994) is the patron saint of gout sufferers, having been thought to advise use of the plant to treat the condition. His dates indicate that ground elder was used for gout long before the monasteries.

John Gerard in 1597 complained of ground elder's invasive habit in his Holborn flower garden. And a lot of present-day gardeners will be wincing at the idea of ground elder as it is so difficult to remove from your garden once there.

But I invite you in your recoiling and shying away to look again and see this plant as food and preventative medicine.

Other than for treating gout and arthritis, ground elder was used as a wound herb, for soothing burns, stings, bites and wounds externally. The German herbalist Tabernaemontanus (1520–1590) used to cook the plant in wine for external uses. Sometimes it was combined with comfrey to make a first aid ointment.

In 2014 Tovchiga et al. in the Ukraine did a trial with ground elder tincture in rats to see if there were uric acid metabolism changes and the suppression of inflammation. The results showed protective action for kidney function and for protecting the liver from carbon tetrachloride-induced hepatitis. Hypoglycaemic properties were also confirmed.

A paper in 2007 showed that mature ground elder flowers contain falcarindiol, with proven COX-1 activity.

Cautions
Only use the young leaves and not to be used after the plant has flowered.

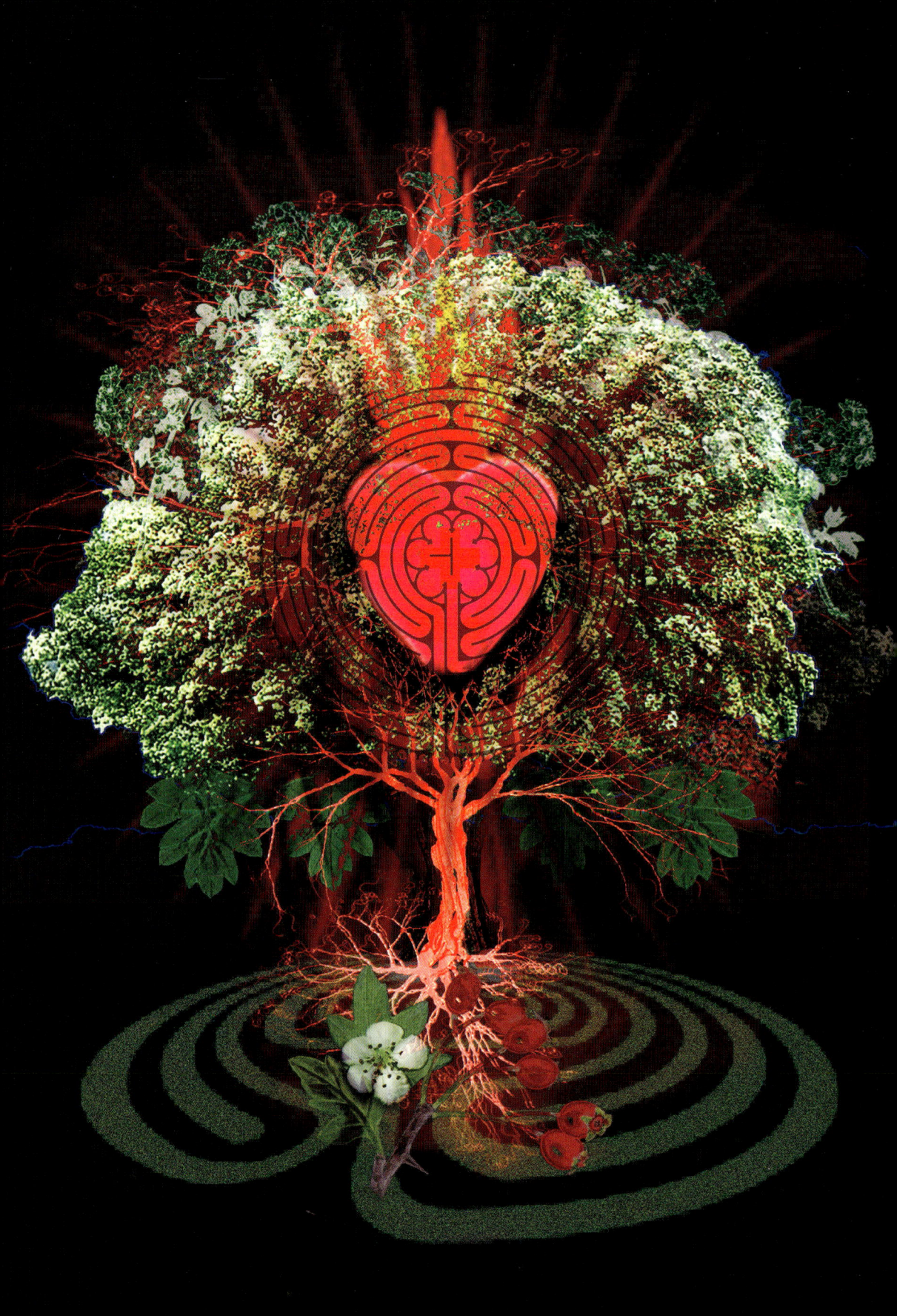

Hawthorn

Crataegus spp.

Gaelic names: Uath; Droigheann

Rosaceae

Parts used – leaf, flower and fruit

I love hawthorn. I love watching it come to life in the Spring, with its leaf buds often with a few of the previous year's berries hanging on. I can't resist a nibble on a few of the first few young leaves. I have used hawthorn for years in clinic and have seen many great results with it.

Hawthorn is in the Ogham and it is the heralder of Summer, the first day of Summer occurring when the hawthorn flowered. This was usually 1 May, Beltaine, but nature does not stick with our calendar and is not always on that day. In any event we can keep within the seasons and that rhythm by watching our local hawthorn and seeing when the flowers start to open.

A few years back we had a cold May, and in Braemar the hawthorn didn't flower until the first few days of June. It's these markers of the seasons and our environment that help me stay in tune with nature a bit more.

The common name mother of the heart is so very apt for hawthorn. It helps regulate the heartbeat. If the heart is running too fast it will help slow it down and if it is a tad sluggish it will pep it up. These qualities are called positively ionotrophic and negatively ionotrophic respectively. Taking hawthorn therefore can help with blood pressure.

I once had a walk with a lady who was really drawn to hawthorn. She hadn't spent much time around plants before and didn't know hawthorn as such. I casually asked her if there had been any heart issues in her family, and she immediately started to well up and tears formed. She turned to me and said her Dad recently had a heart attack.

I explained what hawthorn is good for, and she was quite amazed and started to see the world in a different way. She was almost shocked to learn she had been so drawn to a plant that is good for heart conditions. I explained that she had an intuition for hawthorn, and while we all have intuition modern life and the digital age make it a quieter voice in a lot of people. At the end of the walk we hugged for a long time, and I really hope she now knows she can listen to her own perceptions. That was a deep and meaningful encounter for both of us.

Hawthorn is a good example of synergy, which is when the sum of the parts work but we don't know which isolated compound is the effective one – it is all of them working together.

Hawthorn contains flavonoids and procyanidins. It has a role in calcium metabolism, which increases potassium levels, and acts as an antagonist for the negative ionotrophic action. It improves the existing output of the heart. By increasing blood flow through the coronary arteries and dilation of these arteries it works to improve the coronary circulation.

Therefore it is useful for an aging heart and for helping improve the nutrition available to the heart.

It has been shown to have a mild sedative effect, which is useful if heart issues arise from a nervous origin.

Hawthorn is usually well tolerated and does not accumulate, unlike other heart treatments like digitalis. I'm still wary to give it to patients taking other heart medications as such close monitoring needs to be done. Hawthorn needs time to work properly, and it can be three months or more before the results start to show.

The classic authors Discorides and Galen didn't mention hawthorn. In fact it was little known until the 16th and 17th centuries where the berries are suggested for treating diarrhoea and taken in wine for heart conditions. Goris and Liot in *Pharmacie Galénique* (1942) mention the non-toxic and nonaccumulative effects from a tincture of hawthorn flowers when given as a tonic to reduce heart palpitations and conditions of fear.

It seems it was the Eclectics of late 19th-century America who were the most responsible for hawthorn becoming known as a heart herb. Dr Jennings of Chicago wrote an article on hawthorn as a major heart remedy in 1896. The plant was included in the American *Materia Medica* in 1898. William Fernie wrote in 1897, 'Haws when dried, make an infusion which acts on the kidneys; they are astringent, and serve as well as the flowers, in decoction, to cure a sore throat.'

In Victorian times a Dr Green of County Clare, Ireland mainly treated heart conditions but never divulged his secret. On his passing his daughter revealed in 1894 that he had used a tincture of ripe hawthorn berries.

I do wonder if we only sought out hawthorn when heart issues became more prevalent in the world. Was it because we had more stresses and strains in our day-to-day life?

It is sometimes said that Christ's crown was made of hawthorn. The burning bush Moses saw was also claimed to be a hawthorn.

Some hawthorn trees growing next to wells are covered in pieces of material, beads and other amulets. The 'rag trees' are considered to be places for healing.

A lone hawthorn tree is associated with the Fae and the spirit world; bad luck is associated with anyone that cuts them down. Rituals for healing with hawthorn include for ringworm, sprained ankles and shingles.

Beltaine is linked with fertility and life and death. The smell of the flowers that appear at this time is supposed to resemble semen or rotting flesh, depending on where you read it. Smell is such an interesting topic. What do you smell when you smell hawthorn flowers? You actually are smelling trimethylamine, the chemical responsible.

Hawthorn flowers are not meant to be brought into the house.

Walking sticks are made from the wood. In Holland and Belgium the fresh berries were mixed with flour and made into bread.

Wines, jellies and jams were traditionally made from hawthorn berries. This is partly related to the high pectin content of the berries.

Cautions

Please do not use large doses of hawthorn if you are already on heart medication. Only do this if being closely supervised by a medical herbalist.

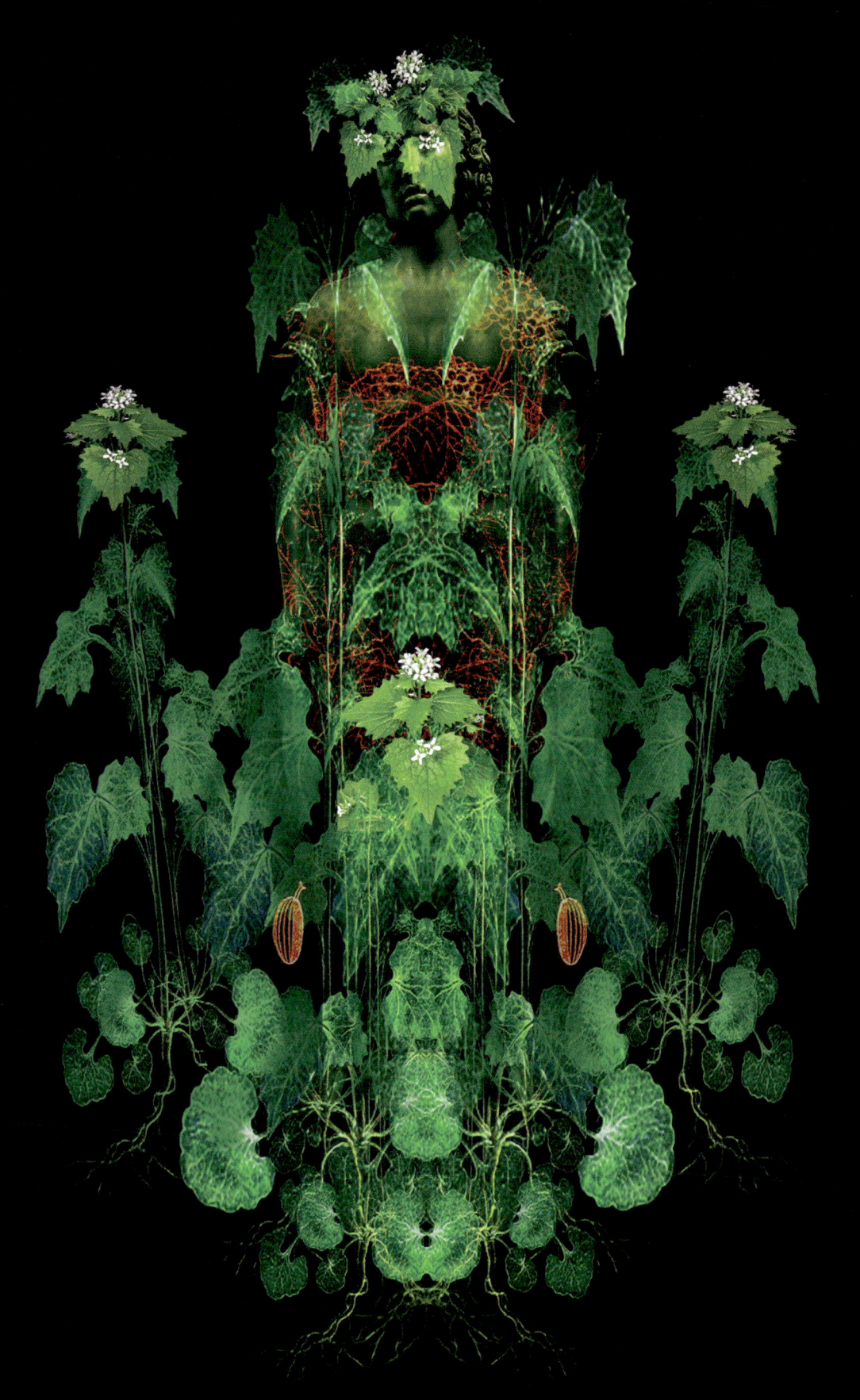

Jack by the hedge

Alliaria petiolata

Gaelic name: Garbhraitheach

Brassicaceae

Parts used: leaves, flowers and seeds

Jack by the hedge is a plant that comes up early in the Spring and lasts until late Autumn. It's a welcome sight that promises bursting flavours, packing a strong and powerful punch. It is absolutely delicious shredded in salads, and is best eaten raw as it loses much of its flavour with cooking and heat. Or, if you prefer its powerful flavours muted, cooking will do this.

As a culinary plant it is great, early in the season before it flowers is the best time.

It has another common name of garlic mustard. This reflects its changing tastes: when young it is more garlic and as it gets older the mustard flavour starts to be more pronounced. The flowers and seeds can be eaten as well, and are almost all mustard flavour, especially the seeds.

Adding it to creamy mayonnaise means its strong flavours are slightly muted and carry well in the oil of the mayonnaise.

My first encounter with this plant was seeing it at the side of the road, initially from the car then as I walking on the South Deeside road. So I went home with a sample of it and looked it up in several books. How had I gone so long not knowing there was another plant tasting of garlic living so close? I love garlic!

Later that day I was going to visit a friend, Eleanor Brown. Eleanor has been a good friend for a long time and she really knows her plants and mushrooms. I walked to her house and noted the few patches of Jack in the hedge along the way so I could discuss the plant and its local locations with her. It was a lovely sunny day and Eleanor was outside getting clothes out and getting wood in – the evenings were still a bit nippy. As I approached her house I saw a patch of Jack by the hedge by her garden. I literally did a small jump for joy as there is no better way to know a plant than to see it growing. There was also no need to travel to find it so we discussed it while looking at it and nibbling. Eleanor also didn't know it either, which made me feel a bit better.

I used to have an insecurity about having to know every plant as you'd need so many lifetimes to cover them all. Instead I started diving deeply into plants I already knew and loved. We did a deep plunge that day into Jack by the hedge, making sure I had identified it properly first, then its safety, its uses and folklore.

Since that time I have nibbled it and made a few dishes with it, taught about it. Teaching teaches you so much, especially when you can listen. On a walk a couple of years ago Jack by the hedge knowledge came from a guest talking about how it was viewed in their home in America. What he said really spun my head.

He explained it is classed as an invasive in quite large areas of America, notably the Northwest and Midwest. It emits a chemical that hinders the growth of other plants and takes over an area. This is interesting because I had no idea it causes problems as it goes on happily alongside other plants here and doesn't get out of control.

This is a good example of nature in balance as Jack by the hedge has become part of the ecosystem in the UK, but its relatively recent introduction to America 150 years or more ago means it has yet to find a balance there.

It would be interesting to look at the soil microbiome of the new areas in America and compare these with the soil in the UK as it is thought that the soil microbiomes play a role in how a plant spreads and competes with other plants as well as crowding them out for light and nutrients. It also creates a selective barrier that seedlings are unable to overcome.

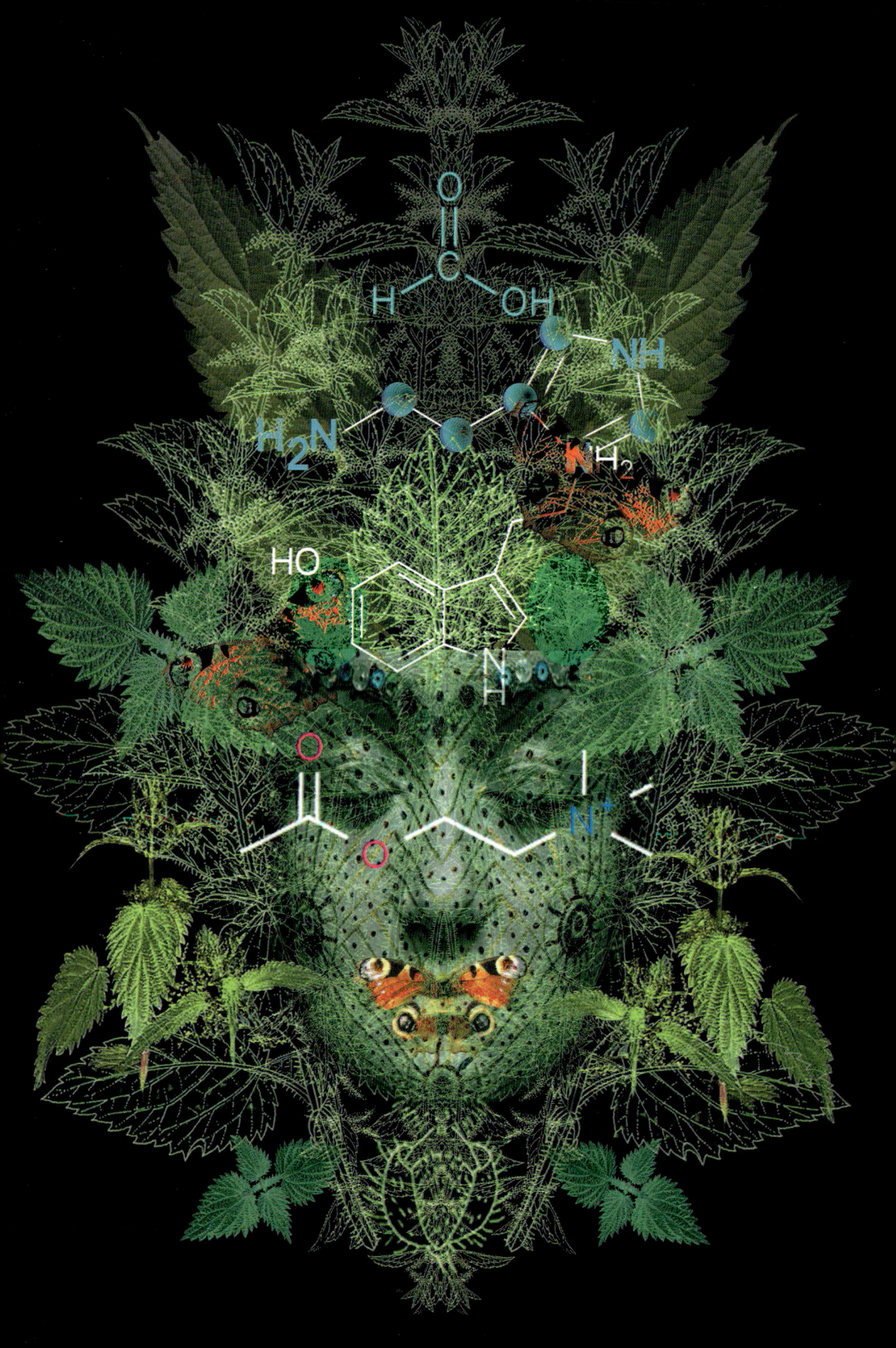

Nettle

Urtica dioica

Gaelic name: Deanntag

Urticaeae

Parts used – young leaf, roots and seed

The stinging hairs of nettle, when examined microscopically, are seen to be hollow tubes composed of silica that resemble glass syringes. When the tips are broken a sharp point is left. The phytochemical soup, the sting, that is injected includes acetylcholine, formic acid, histamine, serotonin and leukotrienes.

The aerial parts of nettle contain flavonoids including rutin, and pretty much every mineral and vitamin you can think of – including iron, magnesium, calcium, potassium, zinc, selenium, and vitamins A, B, C, E and K.

In medicinal properties it is tonic, alterative, astringent, anti-inflammatory, anti-allergy, haemostyptic, diuretic, hypoglycaemic and galactagogue.

Its uses include but are not limited to treatments for anaemia, haemorrhage, skin conditions, joint issues and, interestingly, as a counter-irritant externally for arthritic pain.

W.T. Fernie's *Herbal Simples* (1897) reflects on the legend that Roman soldiers brought nettle seeds to Britain to plant for use as a blood warmer: 'they bethought them to provide Nettles wherewith to chafe their limbs when "stiffe and much benumbed"'.

Nettle leaf stimulates digestion, reduces lethargy and clears phlegm. It is a superb nourisher – it nourishes the blood, which is useful in anaemia; it nourishes the bones and connective tissues; and it nourishes the immune system.

The root contains phytosterols, which help in treatment of BPH (benign prostatic hyperplasia).

Nettle seed has only recently come back into use, for example for kidney function, with American herbalist David Winston a strong advocate.

Nettle soup in the past has sustained many of people. If you ask older folk they tend not to admit using nettles, which were associated with poverty and backwardness. It now feels like the direct opposite, with plenty of restaurants offering a nettle soup on the menu.

Nettles can be eaten as you would spinach or cabbage, and in Scotland they can be an ingredient of haggis.

The Scottish poet Thomas Campbell (1777–1844) said: 'I have eaten nettles, I have slept in nettle sheets, I have dined off a nettle tablecloth. The stalks of the old nettles are as good as flax for making cloth. I have heard my mother say that she thought nettle cloth more durable than any other species of linen.'

In Hans Christian Andersen's tale 'The Wild Swan' a princess had to weave 11 nettle shirts in order to break a spell that had been cast over her 11 brothers, which turned them into swans. She endured painful blistering from the nettles to achieve her task – in real life, it is estimated that it takes 88 pounds of nettles to make one shirt.

Military clothes and uniforms have been made of nettle cloth, while its green dye helped to camouflage the uniforms.

When there have been food shortages people turn to nettles. Martin Martin in 1703 recorded that nettle leaves added to meat or lentil broth were believed to help arthritis. On the isle of Lewis nettles were fermented with reeds to produce an expectorant.

Cautions

Do not eat the leaves of nettle after it starts to flower as it contains microscopic calcium carbonate that can build up and damage your urethra and eventually the kidneys. Stick to young leaves and seeds.

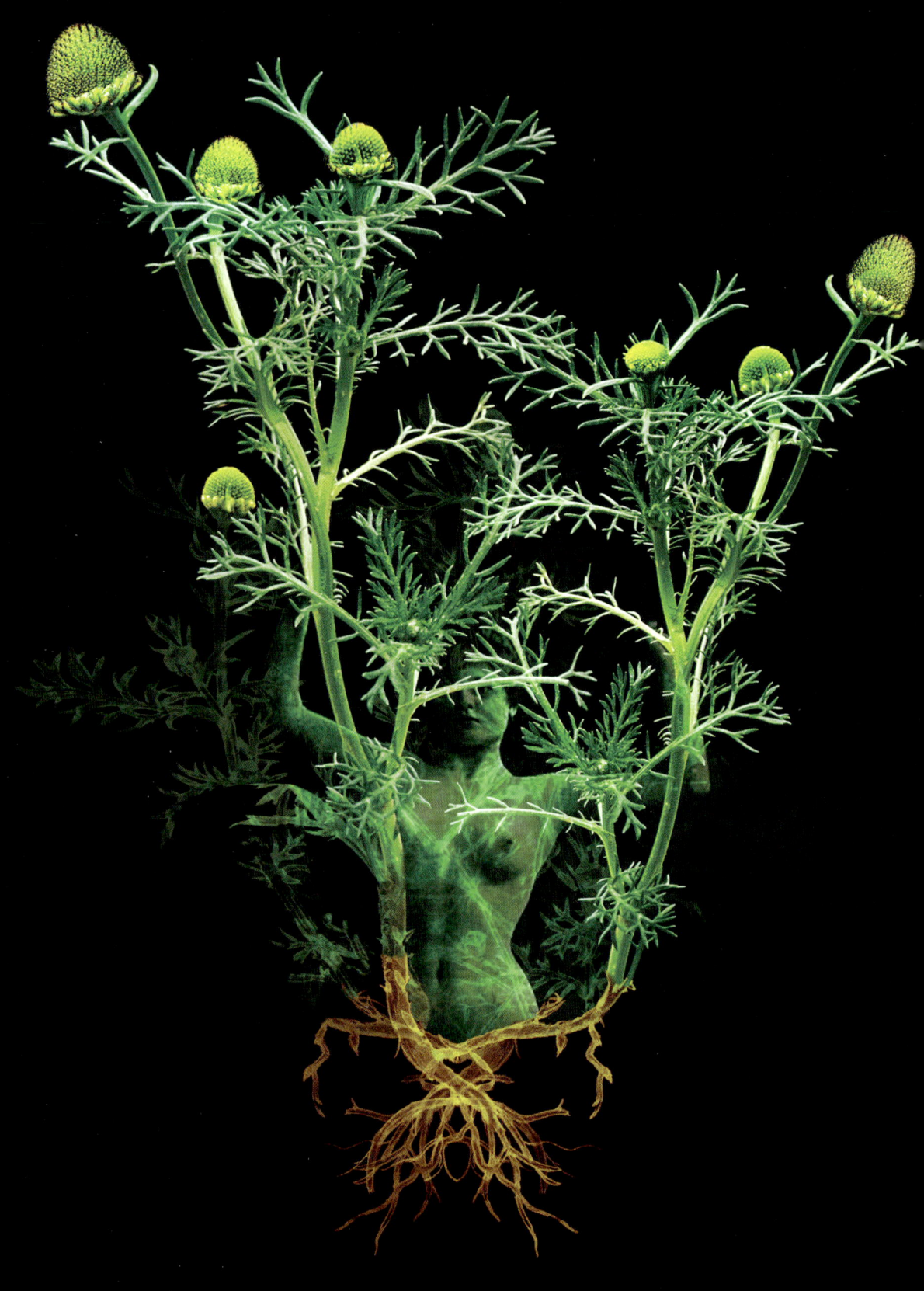

Pineapple mayweed

Matricaria discoidea

Gaelic name: Lus Anainn

Asteraceae

Parts used – aerial parts

Pineapple mayweed is related to German chamomile, *Matricaria recutita*, but does not produce the same blue essential oil. Its own essential oil is green and is made from the flowerheads. This oil reduces anxiety and stress, and is antispasmodic.

It has a vermifugal effect on roundworms, threadworms and whipworms. Made of the aerial parts and taken twice daily, the oil is not as strong as tansy or wormwood.

This marvellous-tasting plant likes to grow along paths and roads. It really does taste of pineapple along with other flavours.

Cautions

None known.

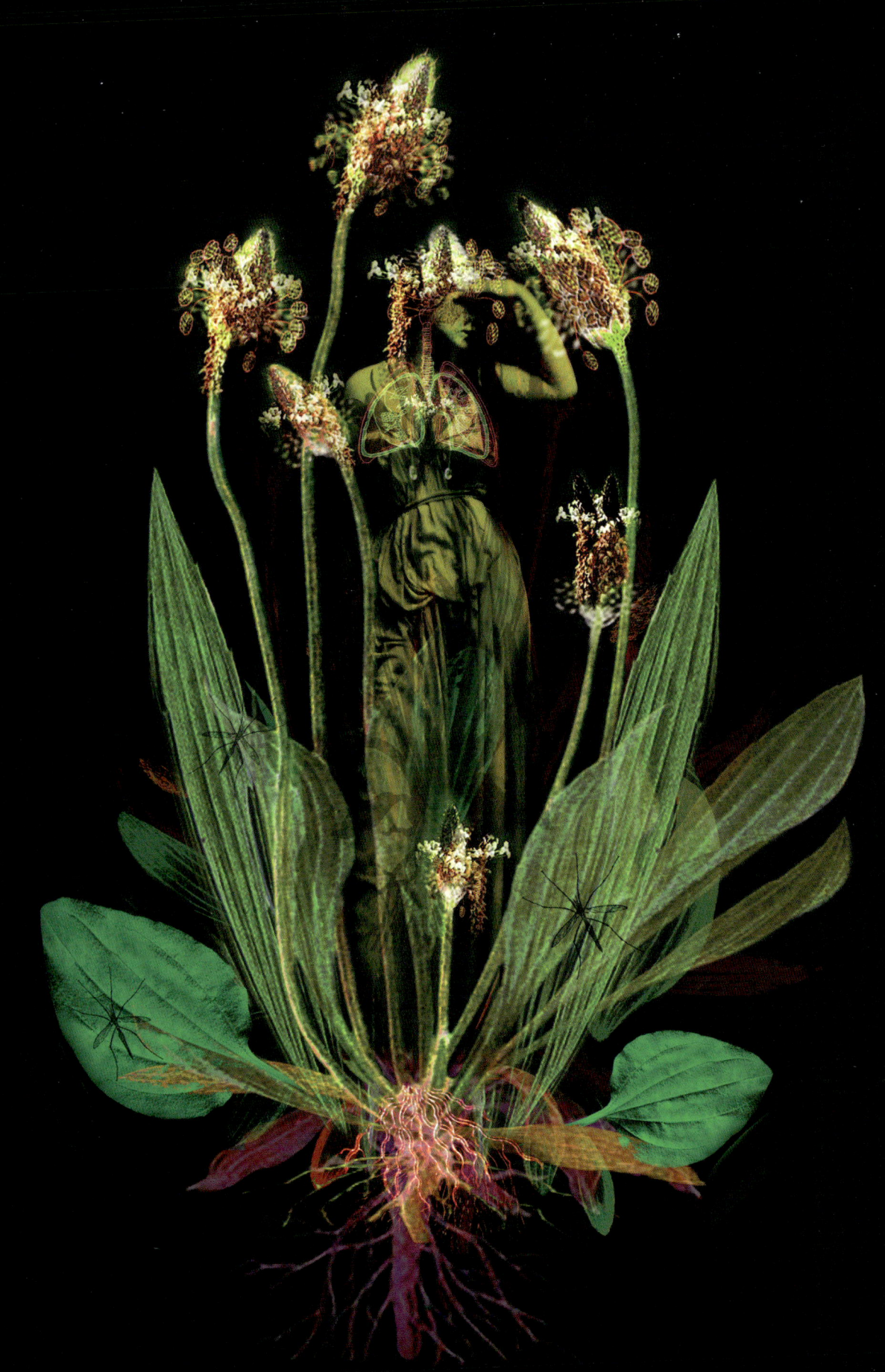

Plantain

Plantago lanceolata and *P. major*

Gaelic names: Ribwort plantain: Slàn-lus. Greater plantain: Cuach Phàdraig

Plantaginaceae

Parts used – leaf and seed

Plantain leaves contain mucilage, tannins, zinc, silica and glycosides. One of its glycosides is aucubin, which has been found to be hepatoprotective.

Plantain has been used as a demulcent, astringent, expectorant, anti-catarrhal, anti-haemorrhage, antiseptic, vulnerary, styptic, antihistamine and as a bulking agent laxative. It is a mucous membrane tonic, with an affinity for the respiratory and gastrointestinal systems.

In the Netherlands equal parts plantain leaves and honey are used as a cough syrup. In New Zealand the Maori set up steam baths with the leaves for treating haemorrhoids.

Plantain is useful for allergic reactions and good for eye issues.

In Scotland, the seeds were used to supplement flour and contain B vitamins.

Some two thousand years ago Pliny the Elder reported that if pieces of flesh were put in a jar and boiled with plantain leaves it would bring them back together again.

Plantain is also good for insect bites, even for midge bites. A few years ago I took out some journalists, and one of the gentlemen had been bitten all around his eyes by midges. I picked a few leaves a plantain and crushed them up between my fingers and handed them to him. He gratefully put them on the bites. By the time we had got back to the hotel the redness had disappeared. I would say it took about an hour.

On another walk with a family the eldest son loved herbal medicine and was keen to learn and understand more. We had a great time. I had explained the story of the journalist and how quick it was for the midge bites to heal, and said plantain can also be used for nettle stings. His younger brother got stung by a nettle. The elder one jumped in immediately with some plantain leaves, crushing them up as he walked. He gave them to his brother who gratefully applied them and after a while said they were working.

When you chew young plantain leaves there are times when they taste of button mushrooms. In the early years of taking people out for walks someone suggested this to me, and, sure enough, we found plantain leaves that taste of mushrooms. This of course fascinated me and I started to investigate. I did not expect to find what I did.

It turns out the taste of mushroom in plantain leaves comes from the mycelium of the snowy wax cap mushroom. The mycelium grows through the leaves, making it an endomycelium. A fair number of plants have these endomycelia.

The snowy waxcap mushroom is an insect-eating mushroom. It goes into the ground and finds insects to eat there. Its mycelium has an enzyme that breaks open the back of the exoskeleton of the insects. When placed on our skin this enzyme helps when we have an insect bite.

It is a practice people have followed for a long time, and now we know why it works – a real intertwinement and interconnection.

Cautions

None known.

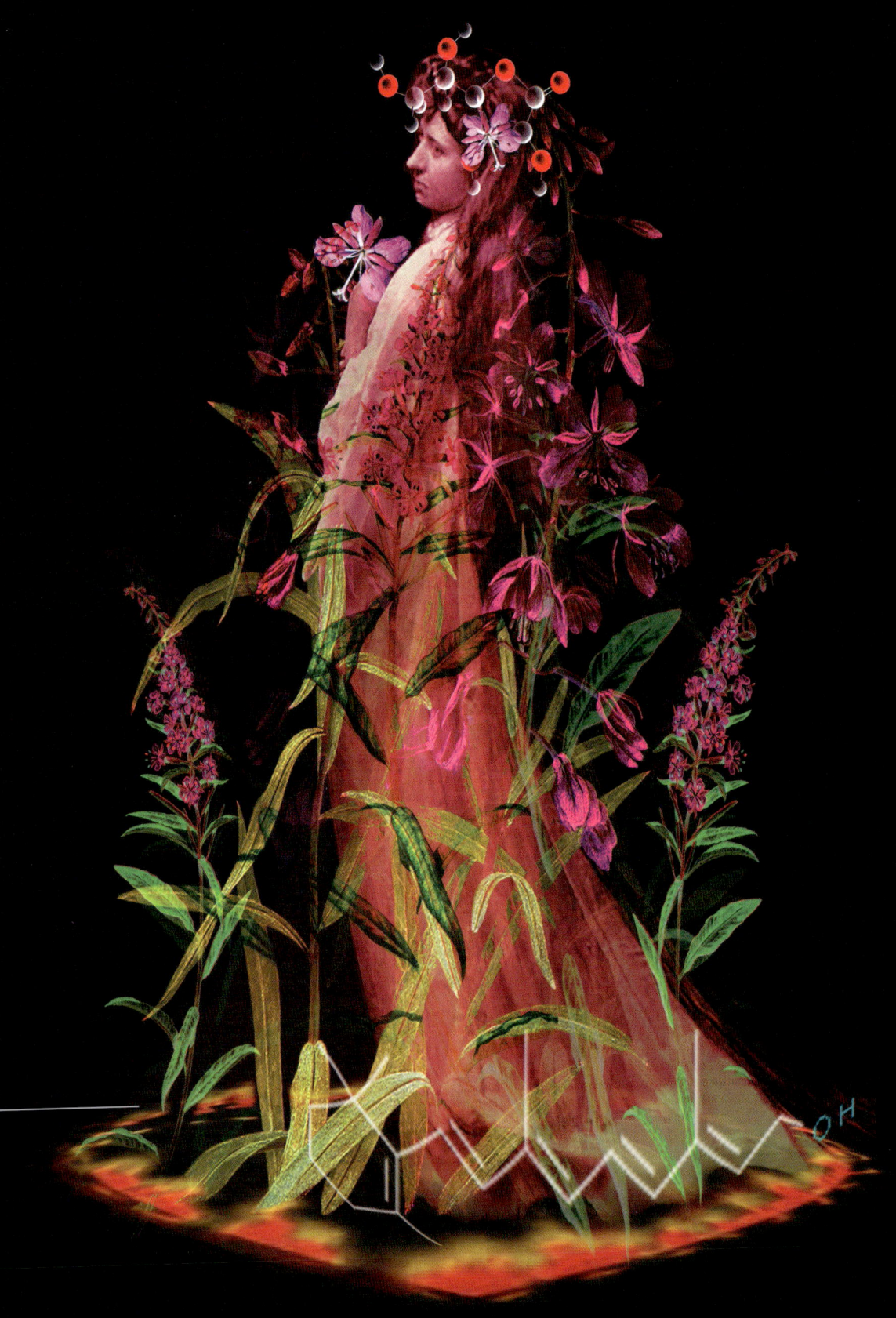

Rosebay willowherb

Chamerion angustifolium

Gaelic name: Seileachan Frangach

Onagraceae

Parts used – young shoots, leaves, flowers and roots

Gerard's *Herball* in 1597 is the first to mention rosebay willowherb in Britain. This tall and striking plant is very noticeable when it is in flower. In grows in large clumps and stands tall, usually along walkways and roads. Its pink flowers give a flash of noticeable colour early in Summer, really standing out against the greens of this time.

It is known as a pioneer plant, which means it comes in first and quickly to any upturned, cleared or disturbed soil. Another name for it is fireweed, for the way it comes up after wild fires. In the Blitz in London in World War Two it often grew after a site had been bombed and gave a welcome splash of colour and flaming beauty, which offered hope.

The seeds are beautifully fluffy and have an amazing aerodynamic ability. They are wind-dispersed with a parachute-type design that is highly effective. Each plant produces around 80,000 seeds. I've watched these seeds being gently blown from the plant, and you see that as one is lifted by the wind it hooks on to the next seed. All in all, it's a very efficient and beautiful form of seed dispersal. These seeds were once used as a free down for bedding and cushions. If you take a few and rub them you will see how soft and silky they are.

One day, after many years of teaching about rosebay willowherb and all its qualities as medicine, tea, food and a condiment, I took out some ladies from Russia. They were excited to see the plant growing in Scotland and immediately told me all about it and how they use it at home. It was reassuringly the same. It always makes me feel good to meet folk who have been brought up with the plants as food and medicine that I'm not so familiar with from my own childhood.

When rosebay stems start to grow in early Spring they are tender. Pan-fried or over a wood fire they make excellent eating. They taste like asparagus, with a texture similar to okra.

The leaves can be made into a tea. They contain a fair amount of tannin and can be a substitute for black tea but without the caffeine. They also contain mucilage, pectin, flavones, and vitamins A and C.

A traditional rosebay tea has been made in Russia for a very long time, often mixed with rose petals. The rosebay leaves are rolled by hand and then left to oxidise for three to five days; then the rose petals added. In Russia it is called Ivan's Tea – you can find videos on YouTube showing the traditional practice.

In Siberia an alcoholic drink is made using the leaves and fly agaric mushroom. Rosebay leaves are a gastrointestinal relaxant and they help with a possible griping caused by the mushroom. Not one I suggest replicating as fly agaric mushroom has muscimol, known to be a psychoactive.

Rosebay flowers produce a great syrup, which retains the pink colour of the flowers. It is delightfully light and floral, and can then be made into ice cream or sorbet. A jelly made of the flowers is made and sold in parts of Canada, called Fireweed Jelly.

The roots contain the enzyme 5-alpha reductase, which inhibits the aromatase enzyme in the prostrate, therefore reducing the amount of testosterone, the hormone associated with an enlarged prostate. Nettle root also contains same enzyme too and is better known for helping with an enlarged prostate.

There isn't much written about the medicinal uses of rosebay willowherb in Scotland or the rest of Britain. In Europe and North America there are a few uses recorded. It is said to be good for asthma, skin conditions, gut irritations and whooping cough, cuts, grazes and sores. There is one mention of being a sedative and useful for tension headaches, while there are many references to it as an antimicrobial and useful for treating prostasis and candidiasis.

Others say it acts as a digestive relaxant, and is therefore good for IBS and other IBD issues. Modern research showing demulcent and astringency properties attest to this.

In logging areas such as in Canada bee keepers follow the logging as fireweed appears. The flowers are a source of food for the bees, and you can buy fireweed honey in some places.

Cautions

The only caution with Rosebay willowherb is a possibility of suffering hayfever from the pollen.

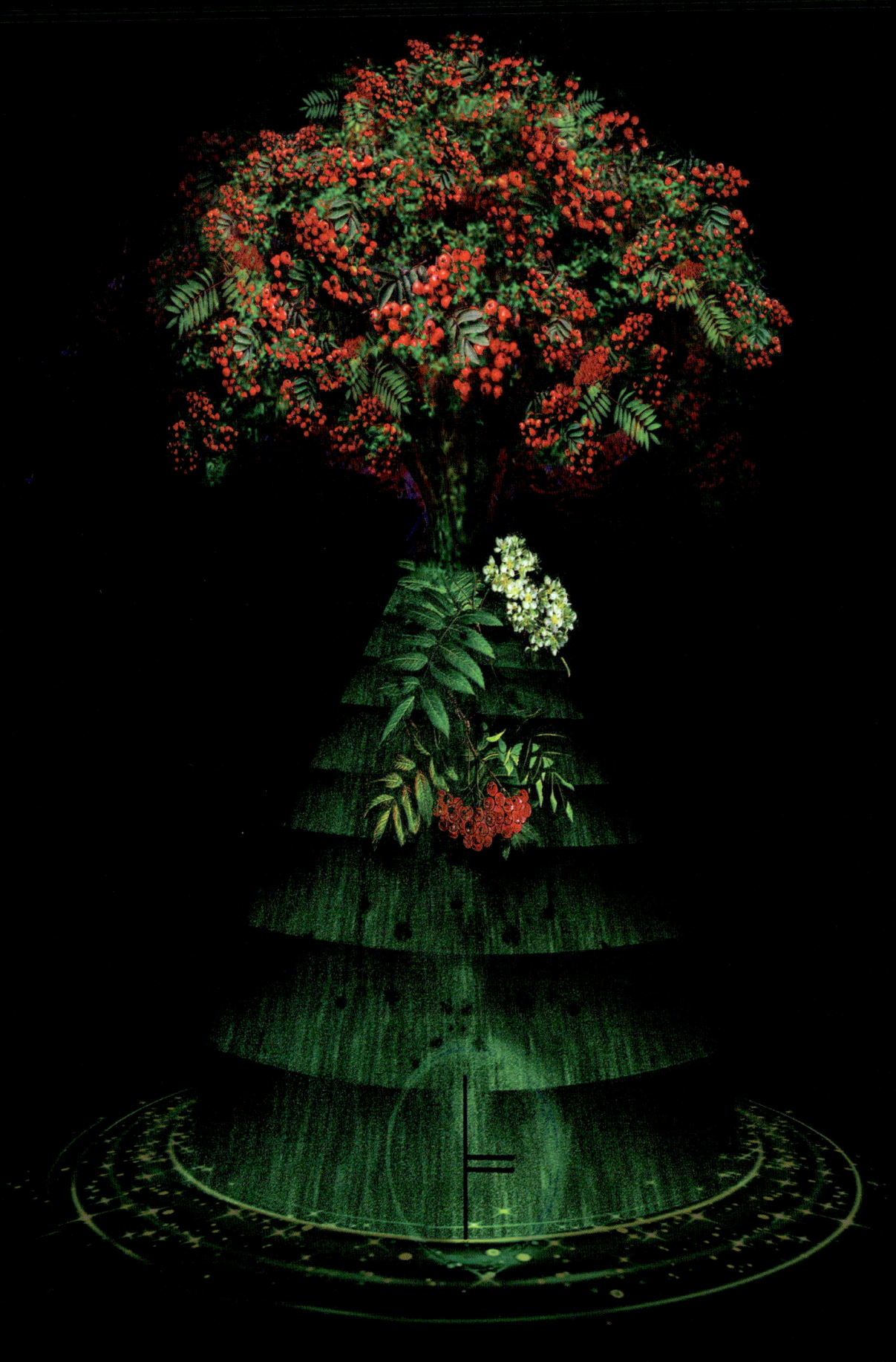

Rowan or Mountain ash

Sorbus aucuparia

Gaelic name: Caorann

Rosaceae

Parts used – fruit

The Rowan tree is a wonderful sight in May and in September, initially for its creamy, white blossoms and then later in the year for its orange/red berries. It is the berries that we forage for, and they make a wonderful tart jelly. It goes well with game meats, strong cheeses and pickles. It's a traditional jelly of Scotland.

If you have tried it then you will know rowan has a flavour that almost hits the back of your throat. That flavour is from the sorbic acid present in the berries. Please be aware you need to boil or freeze the berries before you use them. Before being frozen or boiled the berries contain parasorbic acid, which is not great over a period of time for your kidneys. Don't chance it or be lazy with these berries: always boil or freeze them. The birds do not eat rowan berries before a frost and then almost seem to strip the trees overnight.

In the medieval Irish story 'The Pursuit of Diarmuid and Gráinne', Gráinne asks, 'What are these berries that Finn wants so badly?' Diarmuid replies they are those of the rowan tree the people of the Goddess Dana left in the territory of O Fiachraigh. He explains that every berry on that tree had great virtues, that is, each had the intoxication of wine and the satisfaction of old mead. Whosoever ate three of those berries, even if he were a hundred years old, his age would return to ten and twenty years.

Rowan was considered a tree of protection against evil and witchcraft. Doors had either pieces of it in or the whole door was made of it, and it was planted near the boundaries of properties. Children's cradles had pieces of rowan wood worked into the design, and protective necklaces were made for them.

Amulets were given to fishermen to protect them while they are out at sea. Druids held it to be a sacred tree that was heavily associated with warding off evil spirits and witches. The Vikings believed the first woman came from a rowan tree, and another source I found said it was how Thor's wife was created too.

The berries have vitamins C and A. Sorbic acid has been shown to prevent collagen breakdown, so giving some credence to the medieval Irish tale. The berries are also astringent and antimicrobial, and have been used for urinary tract infections, coughs and colds.

As well as the traditional rowan berry jelly in Scotland there are also accounts of wine, beer, a spirit and the berries being added to mead.

Cautions
Just remember to freeze or boil the berries first before using them.

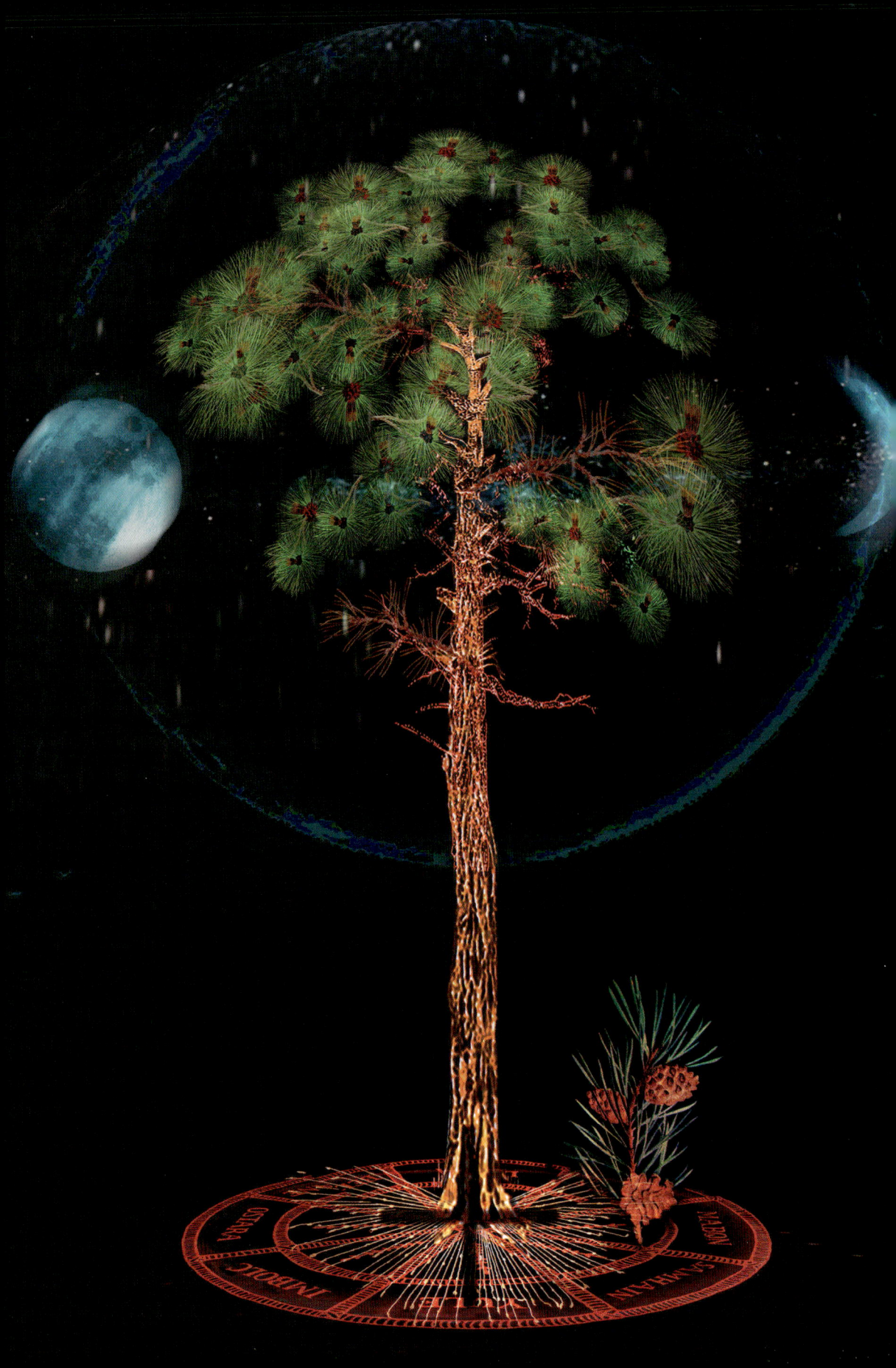

Scots pine

Pinus sylvestris

Gaelic name: Giuthas

Pinaceae

Parts used – needles, cones and bark

Scots pine is symbol of immortality, and warriors' graves were planted with pine. Pine cones are a symbol of male fertility, while in Orkney a lighted pine cone was carried around a new mother to purify her.

Pine resin was used as an antiseptic dressing, and the roots yielded a cough syrup. Pine bark is rich in astringents and was used to treat fevers; pine buds were used for scurvy. An ointment for treating boils resin was made from pine resin mixed with heated pig fat. The astringent tannin rich bark used to treat fevers.

A walk in the world for convalescence to breathe in the pine-fragrant air is part of the reason that tuberculosis sanitaria were established in the Swiss Alps. Pine is known as a respiratory antiseptic.

John Pechey in 1694 wrote: 'The Bark and Leaves cool and bind; wherefore they are good in Dysenteries, and Fluxes of the Courses. A Decoction or Infusion of the Tops in Beer, or some other proper Liquor, is reckon'd very good for the Stone of the Kidnies and Bladder, and for the Scurvy, and Diseases of the Breast. The Nuts have a delicate Taste, and are good for Coughs and Consumptions, and for Heat of Urine. They increase Milk, and provoke Venery.'

The inner bark of the pine was eaten as survival food for Native Americans. In Sweden Linnaeus also reported this same use.

Pine needle tea has a rich vitamin C content and is possibly antiviral.

The original Vicks VapoRub was patented in the US in 1894, and it relied heavily on pine. The current active ingredients are camphor, eucalyptus oil and menthol.

Pine bark also helps stimulate blood circulation owing to its pycnogenol content. Pycnogenol is an oligomeric proanthocyanidin, which are powerful antioxidants. They also protect the collagen in the body, slow the accumulation of fat around the arteries and reduce the risk of heart disease.

Research in 2009 showed that pine polyphenol propanoid polysaccharides inhibit allergic reactions, particularly in asthma.

Earlier findings from 2005 demonstrated that pine was more effective than resveratrol in inhibiting the growth of yeast infections *Candida albicans* and *Saccharomyces cerevisiae*. It was also effective against the bacteria *Staphylococcus aureus*.

Cautions

None known, although some people have an allergic reaction to pine pollen and pine nuts.

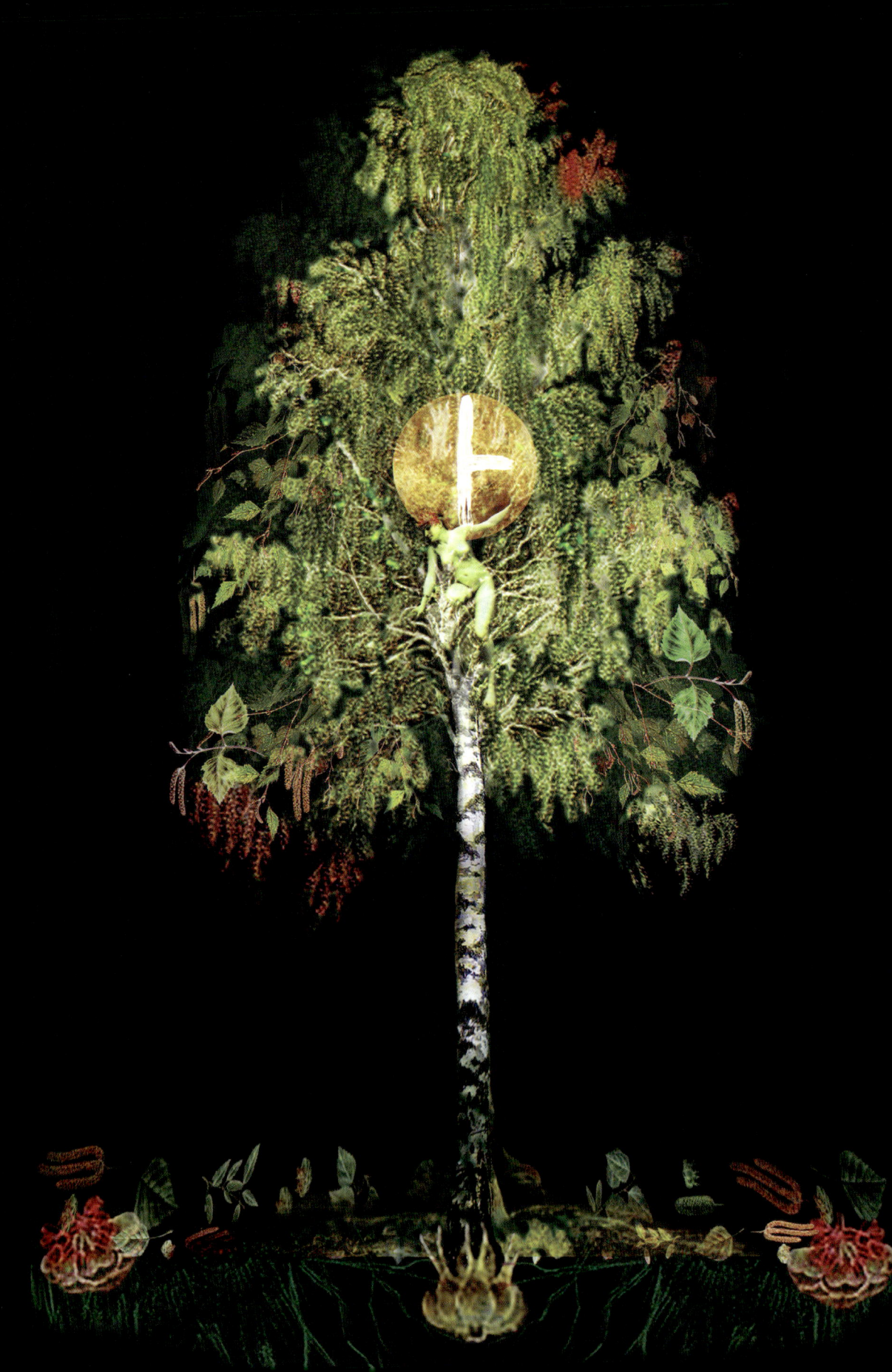

Silver birch

Betula pendula

Gaelic name: Beithe

Betulaceae

Parts used – leaf, sap and bark

The nun Hildegard of Bingen (1098–1179) was the first European to write about the properties of silver birch.

Two hundred years ago the poet Samuel Taylor Coleridge referred to the birch tree as 'the lady at the woods' for its light colour and elegance.

The leaves of silver birch are rich in potassium and are used as a diuretic. They have been shown to help the secretion of uric acid, and are therefore good for gout. They also contain saponins, which can be toxic for some people and shouldn't be ingested for any length of time.

Another use for the leaves is as an anti-inflammatory poultice for easing arthritis. It is highly prized in Russia for this use. The leaves can help promote sweating and therefore reduce fevers.

Birch tar has been used topically for psoriasis and arthritis. It is also commercially valuable in the perfume industry and in toothpastes. It has been useful to make charcoal and to smoke fish; it made birch bark paper, and the wood was made into cotton reels. Brooms or besoms were made from birch twigs.

The betulinic acid in silver birch has been shown to be anti-tumour and useful against skin cancers, human melanomas and brain tumours. It is also been found to suppress HIV.

Birch bark contains salicylates, which are known to be anti-inflammatory. Betulin itself is antifungal, antibacterial and antibiotic.

Birch sap flows at the start of Spring, and as the sap rises in the tree we can tap into it and have some for ourselves as a tonic and preventative for arthritis. It contains potassium and other minerals that in the past we lacked over Winter,

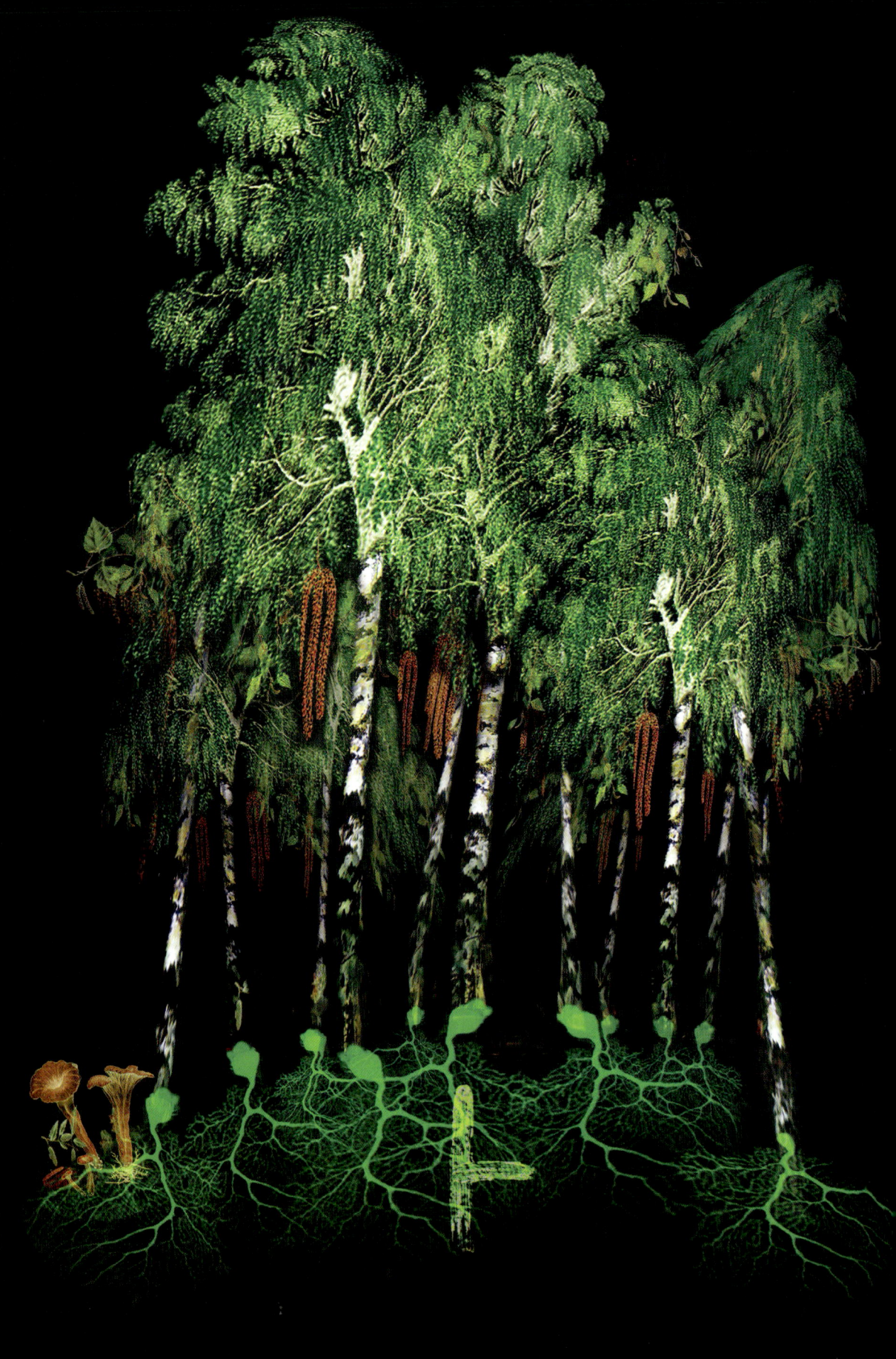

so taking the sap replenished our own bodily stores. It can be drunk straight from the tree, but be aware it goes off very quickly without being stored in a fridge or frozen. It makes a lovely wine, which is a great way to preserve it.

Rolls of birch bark have been found in Mesolithic sites. The name derives from Sanskrit *bhurga*, which means the tree whose bark can be used for writing. In Ireland birch is considered to be disliked by the fairies.

Cautions

None known.

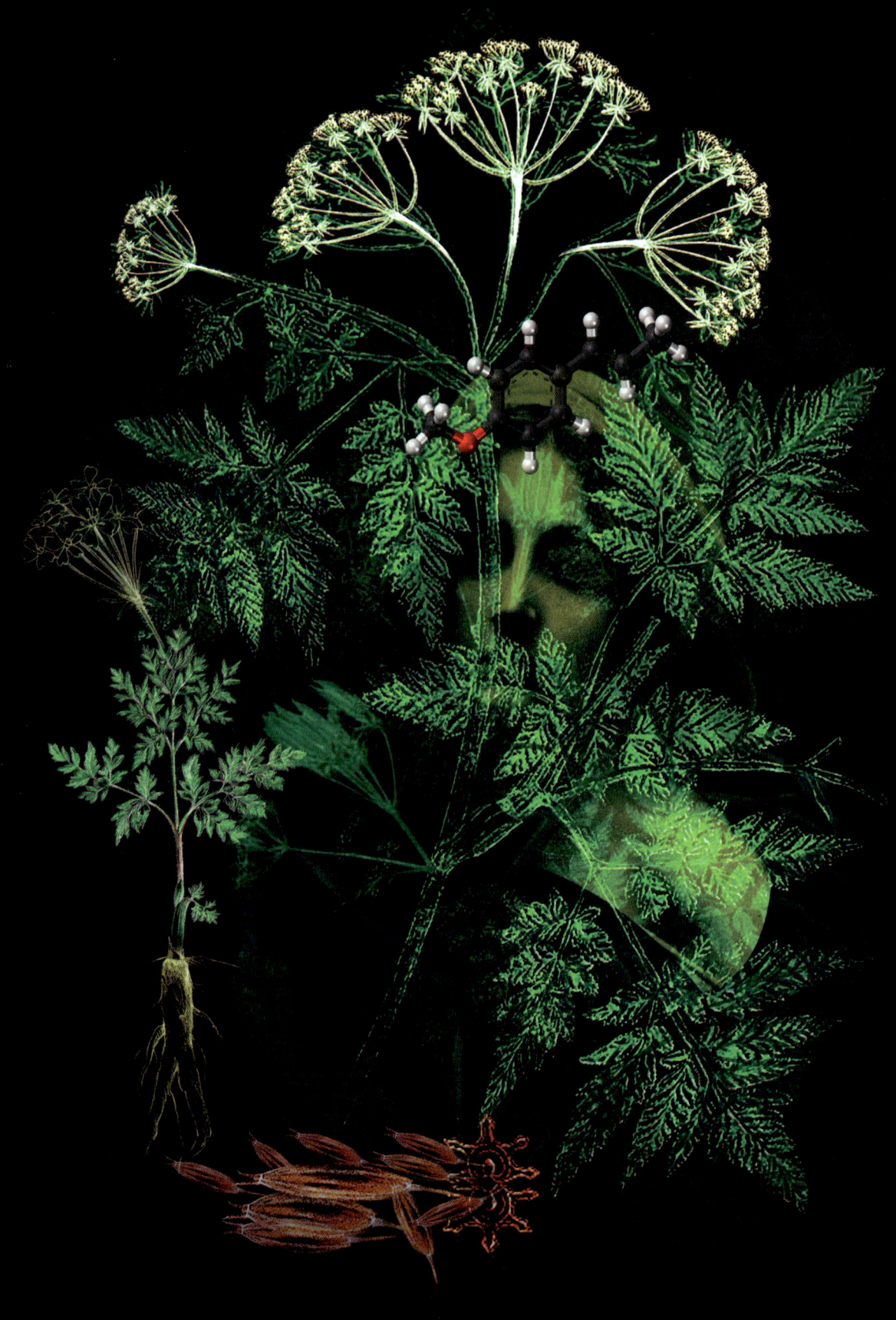

Sweet cicely

Myrrhis odorata

Gaelic name: Cos uisge

Apiaceae

Parts used – leaf, stem, flower and seed

Locally to where I live we have lots of sweet cicely, and the young seeds are often nibbled as folk pass them. This suggests that passed-on knowledge is still important in our modern world, with all its tech and multiple forms of communication, and that word of mouth and oral traditions are still valued – maybe even more so now.

Chatting with your neighbours and folk in your community was so highly welcomed in the lockdowns that we started to realise its value and worth in our lives. Knowledge passed on by a trusted person locally is a very valuable thing indeed. It also highlights the art of listening as one-way communication isn't going to work.

Sweet cicely is a delightful feathery plant often seen growing near water. It has a strong and delightful aniseed scent and taste. Please note that it is really important to not mix up this plant's ID with certain members of the same family, such as hemlock, cowbane and hemlock water dropwort, all of which can kill you.

It is at this point I remind you again do not eat anything you don't know.

The sweet taste of sweet cicely is attributed to the chemical anethole.

Medicinally it can be used as a stomachic, carminative, expectorant and tonic. It is useful to take for coughs, flatulence and anaemia. One source I read said it helps restore vigour and is beneficial for when folk have lost their enthusiasm for life. This is thought to be because it helps digestion and appetite, and improves absorption of nutrients.

Taste-wise, sweet cicely is great with fish and fantastic with rhubarb. It has a long growing season.

Cautions

None known. But please do not get this plant mixed up with other members of the Apiaceae family, which includes hemlock and hemlock water dropwort.

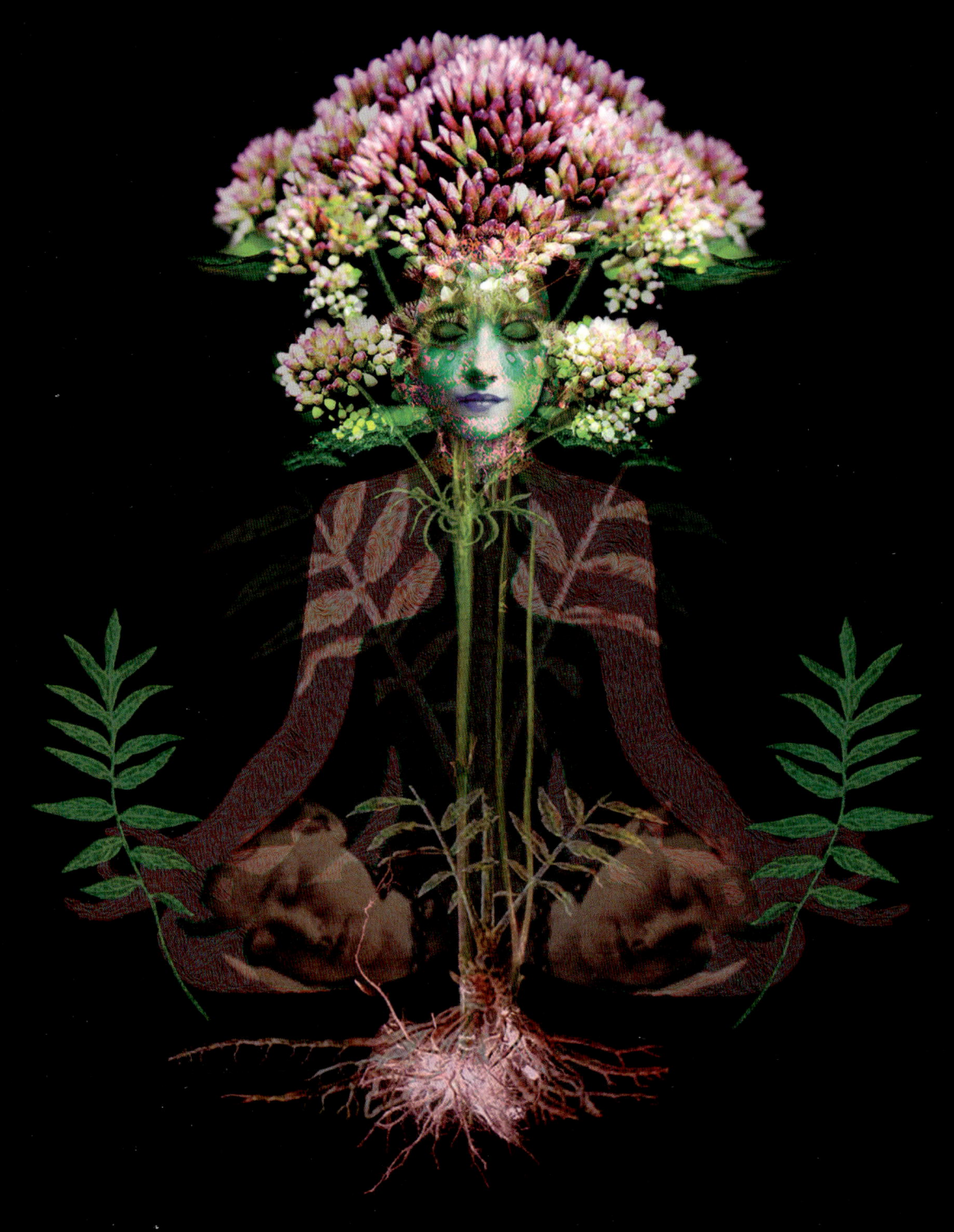

Valerian

Valeriana officinalis

Gaelic names: Lus na Snàthaid; Lus nan trì bilean; Carthan-curaidh

Caprifoliaceae

Parts used – flower and root

This plant is well more well-known than some others in this book, having been available to us in various ways in high street shops and garden centres for a while now. It is often used in commercial herbal sleeping teas and capsules.

I first encountered valerian quite young as my brother was prescribed it, in Germany, for restless sleeping as a young boy. It worked wonderfully for him and we all got a good night's sleep as a result. Valerian was highly prized in our household.

It likes to grow near water courses and rivers, and has a lovely white flower similar in shape and colour to yarrow but with different leaves. As well as different leaves the smell of valerian is what really gives it away. To me when it first blooms it reminds me of jasmine and ylang ylang, and is a delight.

Not long after opening, though, the smell starts to change and, oh boy, does it change. It starts to smell more like the roots, which are the traditionally used part of valerian. It is a smell once known you are unlikely to forget. It permeates a room very well, and you can always tell when I've used it in a herbal mix.

The smell starts to change to what is reminiscent of old socks and male cat pee, which is highly aromatic. Some folk are really drawn to the smell – I've found it is usually these folk that require the benefits of this plant and it suits them well.

Cats love this plant and will seek it out in the same way they look for catnip. In my first year of training we did a module called pharmacosgnosy, which helped us identify the plants and many different levels. We were given small bags of plants to take home to learn from. I put a sample of valerian in a drawer, and one of my cats at the time was found the next day, fast asleep in the drawer surrounded by the open bag of valerian.

Rats also have a fascination with valerian. It is speculated that it may have been this plant in the pocket of the Pied Piper that helped him lead all the rats out of town.

The history of valerian goes back a fair way. Dioscorides mentioned it some two thousand years ago, and in 1592 the Italian botanist Fabio Colonna published findings that claimed that valerian had cured epilepsy. In 1640 John Parkinson wrote about it for headaches, colds and coughs, eye problems and colic, as well as mentioning it as a mild wound healer.

In 1707 John Pechey agreed with Colonna, and in 1772 John Hill published *Valerian, or The Virtues of That Root in Nervous Disorders*. The *American Pharmacopoeia* from 1820 to 1936 listed it as an antispasmodic. The latest *British Herbal Pharmacopoeia*, published in 1996, has it as a sedative.

The name valerian in medieval times was heal-all and derives from Latin *valere*, meaning 'to be well'.

Over 150 compounds have been identified in valerian research but emphasis is being placed on their synergistic effects. The way valepotriates break down into valerianic acid is where research is focused. It has an affinity to the GABA receptors and has been shown to potentiate central nervous system depressants. This would explain its sedative effect. It was used for shell shock in both world wars to the extent that demand outstripped supply.

For some people it has the opposite effect, and when these folk use it as a sleep remedy it can keep them awake. I've known this effect on patients too, and we do not know why this happens but it is worth trying a small amount before recommending it.

Saying that, valerian is worth its weight in gold for those it does work on as a good sedative, antispasmodic, aromatic digestive, anxiolytic, for nervous digestion issues and headaches, particularly tension headaches and migraines. It is good for treating insomnia and hypertension. It known as a grounding herb and therefore useful in panic attacks and to bring harmony back within ourselves.

Its flavour is unusual, and I like to use the young flowers for recipes more than the root. Partly as I don't like digging up roots of plants, I buy in valerian root from cultivated sources.

Cautions
None known, but some people may dislike it intensely.

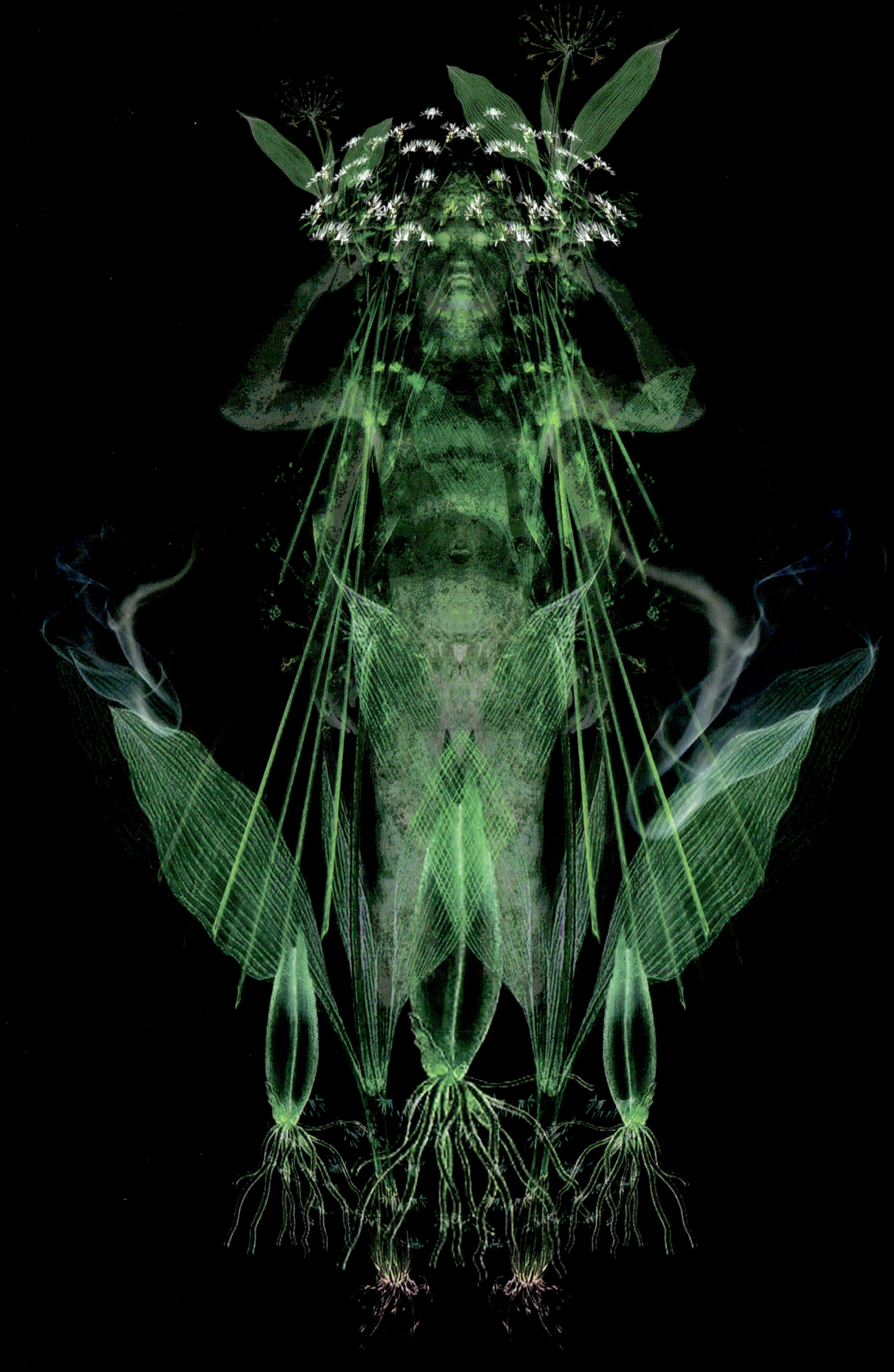

Wild garlic

Allium ursinum

Gaelic name: Creamh

Amaryllidaceae

Parts used – leaf, flower and seed

Wild garlic or ramsons often heralds Spring for a lot of people, and the familiar strong scent of carpets of wild garlic is a delight after Winter. The promise of warmer weather and more plants springing up is such a part of that feeling.

So many people are aware of wild garlic now it's wonderful. They are many recipes on the internet. It felt wrong to leave it out here as it is so iconic and well known. I've included my own favourites recipes.

Wild garlic was not my first plant to identify in the wild. It was nettle when I was a child, then dandelion. When I started to study medicinal plants I set off with those two and worked my way out by identifying the plants growing next to them on the Isle of Lewis, the place I really began to know my plants and get properly familiar with them. Lewis is not an environment known for its areas of woodland. I was used to moors and sea shores. So learning wild garlic took me a while as it was a new environment to understand.

Wild garlic poultices were applied to infected wounds with an infusion used to strengthen the blood. In the world-wide influenza pandemic of 1918 people carried ramsons in their pocket to help ward off the infection. We have no idea if this worked or not.

It has been and can be used as a vegetable and a green sauce made with sorrel for eating with fish.

As wild garlic increases the effect of blood-thinning medication, don't eat too much if you're on such medication.

It is good for digestion and helps reduce blood fats. It also contains allicin, the same as common garlic. It's a diuretic and was traditionally used for kidney stones, coughs, colds and flus, and it also clears mucus. It contains vitamin C.

Cautions
Do not eat too much or it might cause a gastric upset.

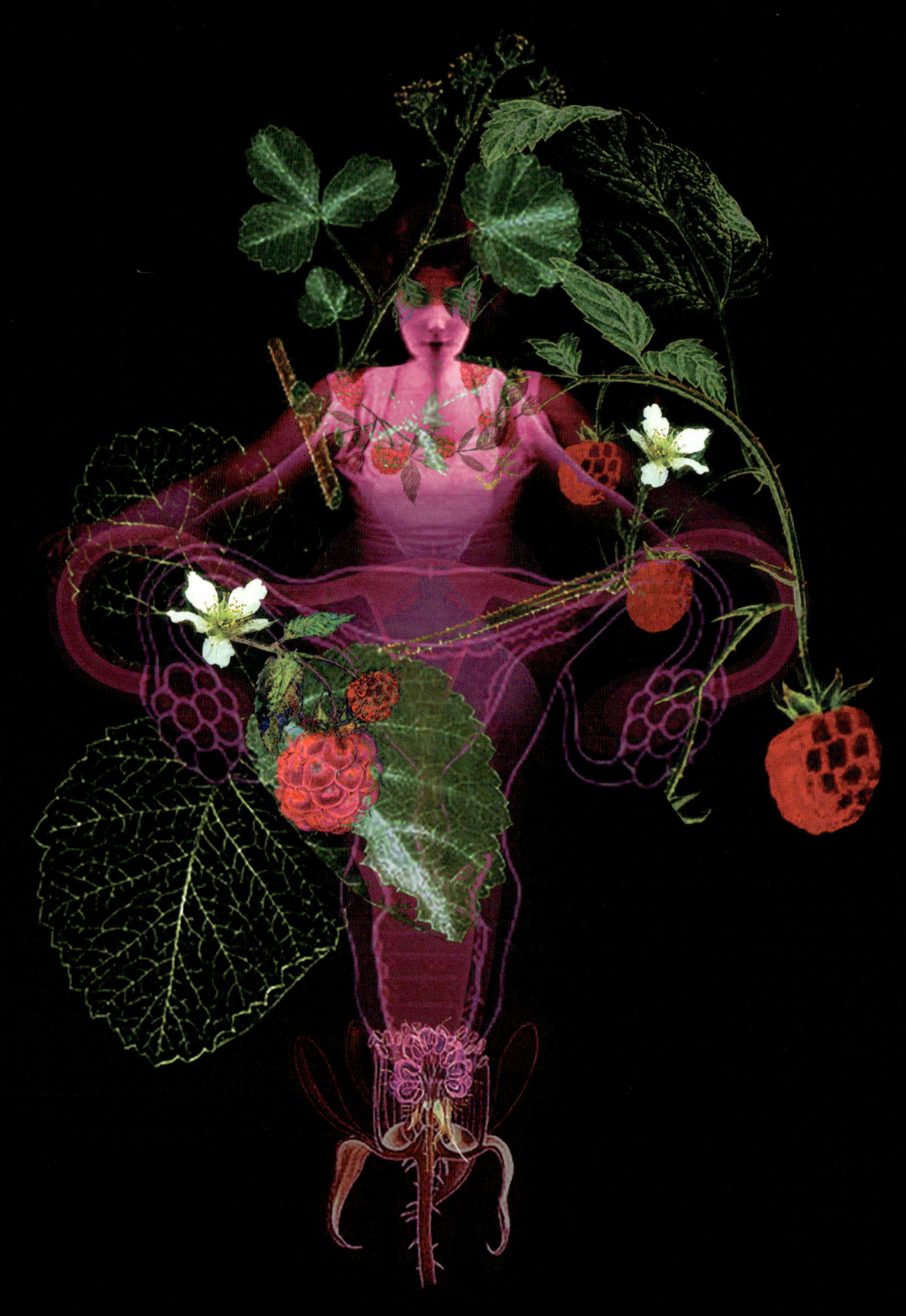

Wild raspberry

Rubus idaeus

Gaelic name: Sùbh-craoibh

Rosaceae

Parts used – leaf and fruit

Wild raspberry has a different flavour than cultivated ones, with a hint of vanilla. For their smaller size they pack a good punch.

The leaves are known for their use as tea in the latter third of pregnancy to strengthen the womb and relax the cervix. This should all be done under the supervision of an experienced herbalist.

The leaf contains calcium, iron, manganese and vitamins A, the Bs and C. The fruit is high in salvestrols. This was the first resveratrol to be discovered, and there are numerus papers on how these help us in our health – they are the main reason we should eat lots of berries.

Tannins in the leaf make them an astringent. In the Highlands they were used for treating wounds, ulcers and for diarrhoea as well as for conjunctivitis.

They are mentioned as far back as Dioscorides some two millennia ago. In 1735 the Irish herbalist K'Eogh used raspberry fruit in honey for eye inflammations, fevers and boils.

My lovely dog Rosie would wait by the wild raspberry canes for permission to eat them. She could barely contain her excitement, running up ahead and waiting till I would signal a yes. She would dive in, so sweet to watch. Guests would love this too.

Rosie was amazing at being well behaved, and I swear she could read people and their emotions way better than most humans and act accordingly. This ability made her behave in the way each person liked.

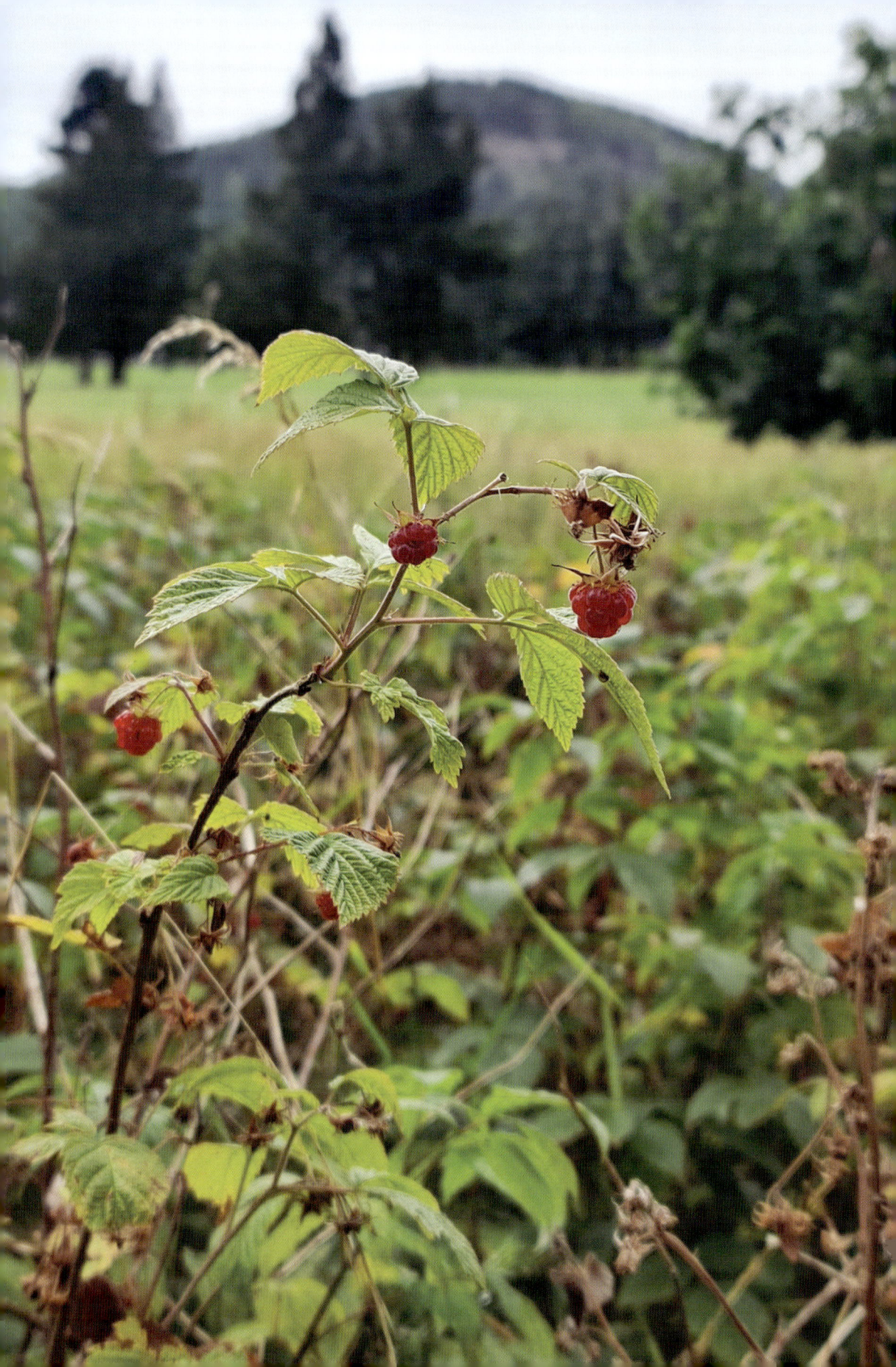

I still miss her, and words are never enough to explain the loss of someone so beautiful in your life. I'm forever grateful that she was part of mine and taught me so much. She loved making people happy and did that for many, many people and creatures. Those reading this that met her will know what I'm talking about and have their own story.

A vinegar of wild raspberry fruit was made in Ireland to help with coughs, and it is great as a salad dressing.

Cautions
Do not take the leaves in pregnancy before the third trimester.

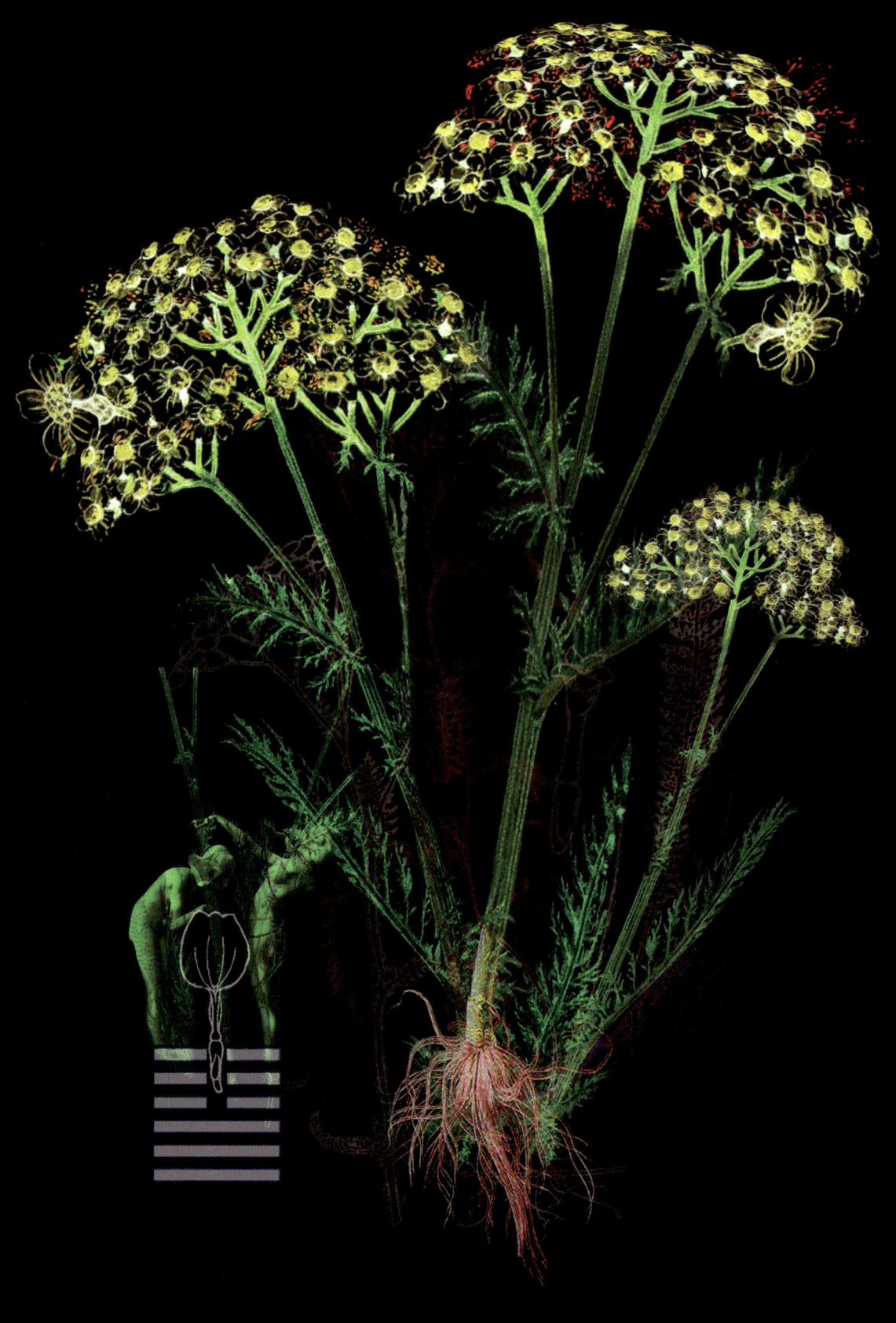

Yarrow

Achillea millefolium

Gaelic name: Lus Chasgadh na Fala

Asteraceae

Parts used – aerial parts

This plant is so fascinating and affects so many areas of the body. It has a very long history of use. A.I. Coffin writes in *A Botanical Guide to Health* (1855), 'There is not a common plant in this country that can be applied more beneficially in the early stages of disease.' Rudolf Weiss's *Herbal Medicine* (1988) says it was used for disorders of the reproductive system and lower abdomen caused by atonic conditions.

Yarrow is used to treat stomach ache in lots of countries, with its bitter principle helping in acute and chronic dyspepsia; it is also an appetiser in anorexia. It is a circulatory stimulant, particularly for the peripheral nervous system. It is a mucous membrane tonic and a diaphoretic, which means it induces sweating. And it has been used as an eyewash for conjunctivitis. Allergic dermatitis has reportedly been helped by it.

In the battle of Troy Achilles is said to have used yarrow to treat his soldiers' bleeding. This reference to Achilles is partly where it gets its Latin name from. Dioscorides knew it, and it kept its importance all through the Middle Ages. I've known it used for toothache. In the first lockdown my teeth fell apart and exposed the nerve. It was the time we couldn't get to a dentist very easily, and so I used paracetamol and yarrow tincture and tea.

I conducted an experiment, and found the yarrow tincture was far better at removing the pain and keeping the pain away for longer than the pharmaceutical.

In the late 19th century Alexander Carmichael collected a song sung by the woman of the Hebrides:

I will pluck the Yarrow fair,
That more benign shall be my face,
That more chaste shall be my speech.
That more sweet shall be my lips,
that more chaste shall be my speech
Be my speech the beams of the sun,
And my lips as sweet as the strawberry.

May I be an Isle in the sea,
May I be a hill on the shore.
May I be a star in the waning moon,
May I be a staff to the weak.
Wound can I every man,
But no man can wound me.

John Lightfoot in 1777 said: 'Highlanders still continued to make an ointment of it, do sometimes thrust a leaf of it up their nostrils to make their nose bleed. Young girls would cut it before sunrise, place it under their pillow and hope to dream of their sweetheart in their dreams. If their back was turned to them it would mean they would not marry but if they were facing them marriage would shortly follow.'

It was hung over doors to keep miss fortune away. In the I Ching, a Chinese divination tool, stalks of yarrow were tossed into the air and the future read from how they landed.

Years ago, when in clinic at Westminster University, I ended up being the only student there, with just a couple of patients. It was unusual to have the qualified practitioner all to yourself, with time to discuss plants not in relation to a patient. So the lovely practitioner decided to help me relax and tune in to the plants.

We quietly sat and she started to help me remove thoughts from my head. There's a lot to think about in a clinic – patients, medicine, setting, personal interactions, getting back to lodgings, what is for lunch – but eventually my thoughts cleared. Then she asked what plant came to mind. Yarrow!

A picture of yarrow was clear and strong. It took me a bit by surprise. I suppose I didn't think this was something that would work but was going along with it. Don't get me wrong. I had times and experiences that made me realise herbal medicine is more than science in its present form. I just wasn't sure how you equate it, put it into words.

I still find it difficult expressing those feelings. All I know is that moment seeing yarrow in my mind's eye and discussing it afterwards made me stronger. I felt I had a wonderful plant ally by my side.

All plants and fungi hold their own and bring so much to the table. Yarrow has been depicted as a warrior, as a strong plant that has many, many uses.

It is diaphoretic, which means it induces sweating, which only happens if there is something for the body to fight, like a virus. It helps stem blood flow, is amazing for toothache and for reducing the tooth decay bacteria of the mouth. Win, win!

It helps open up the capillaries located in feet, hands and head, and this improves circulation. Increasing blood flow around the body takes some load off the heart and can reduce blood pressure.

As with a lot of plants yarrow is anti-inflammatory. It is a wonderful aromatic bitter, and this helps with digestion. There is a huge amount of clinical evidence and thousands of years of written accounts for this plant but still not many scientific papers. So it can get overlooked, and it really shouldn't.

Cautions
None known.

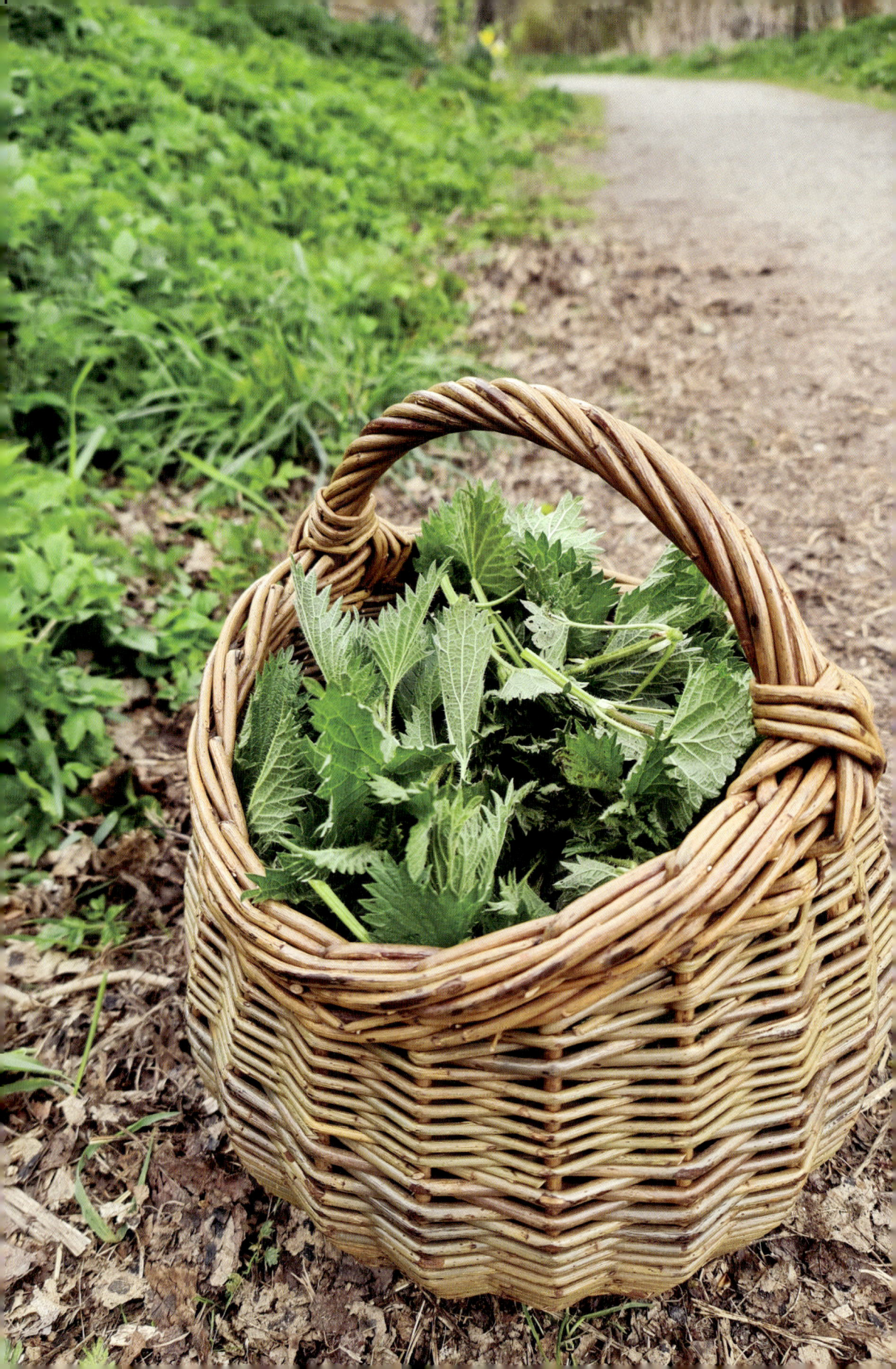

Recipes

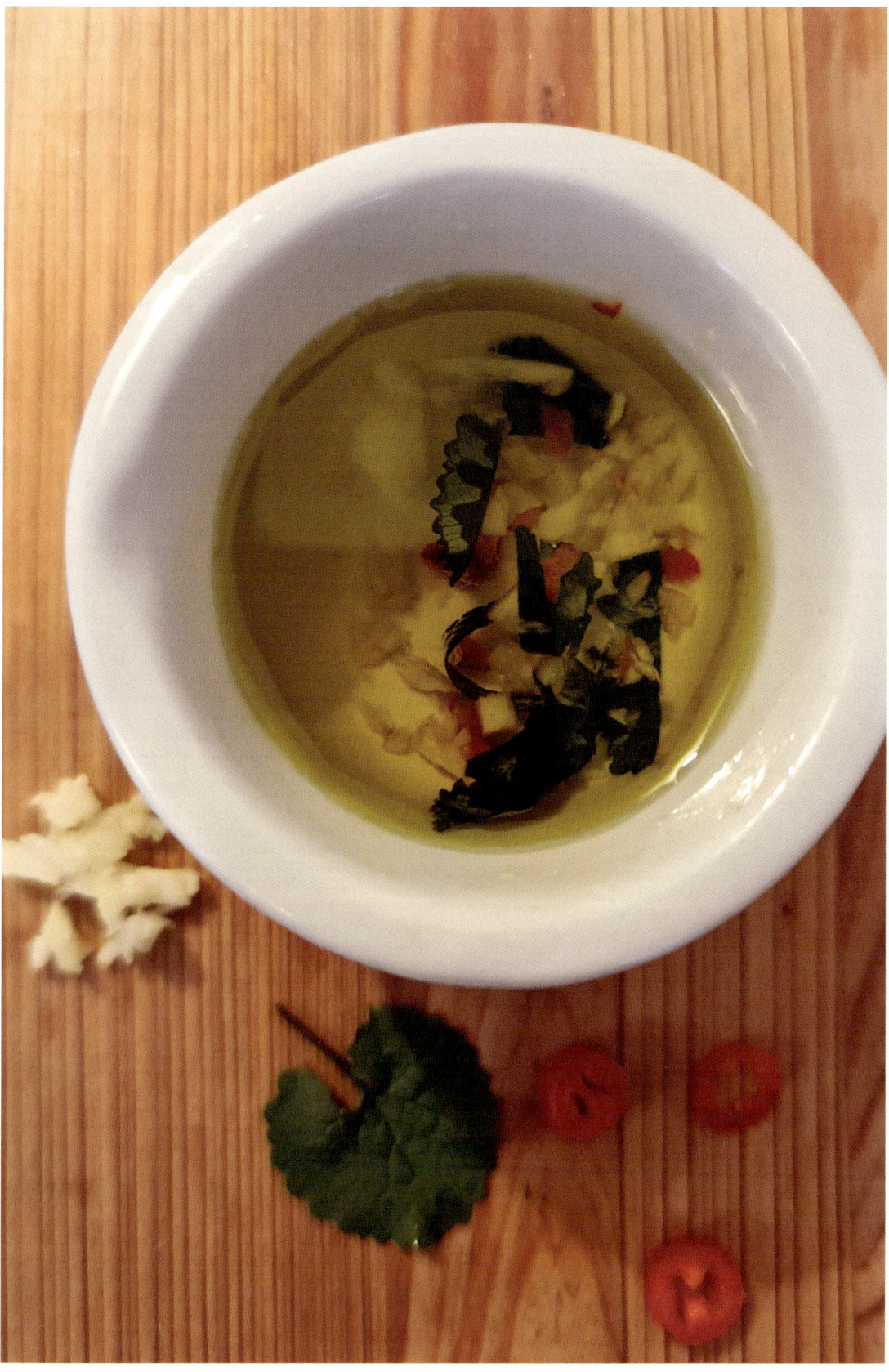

Dipping sauces

Jack by the hedge, chilli and garlic dipping sauce

About 5 medium leaves Jack by the hedge
100ml olive oil
1 chilli, deseeded and chopped finely
1 clove of garlic, crushed and diced

Add the olive oil to a sterilised 300ml jar.

Add all the other ingredients and put the lid on the jar and shake so all the ingredients are coated in the oil. You can use it as it is, but the oil takes on the flavours more over a few days. For me it is best three to five days after making.

Foraged Condiments

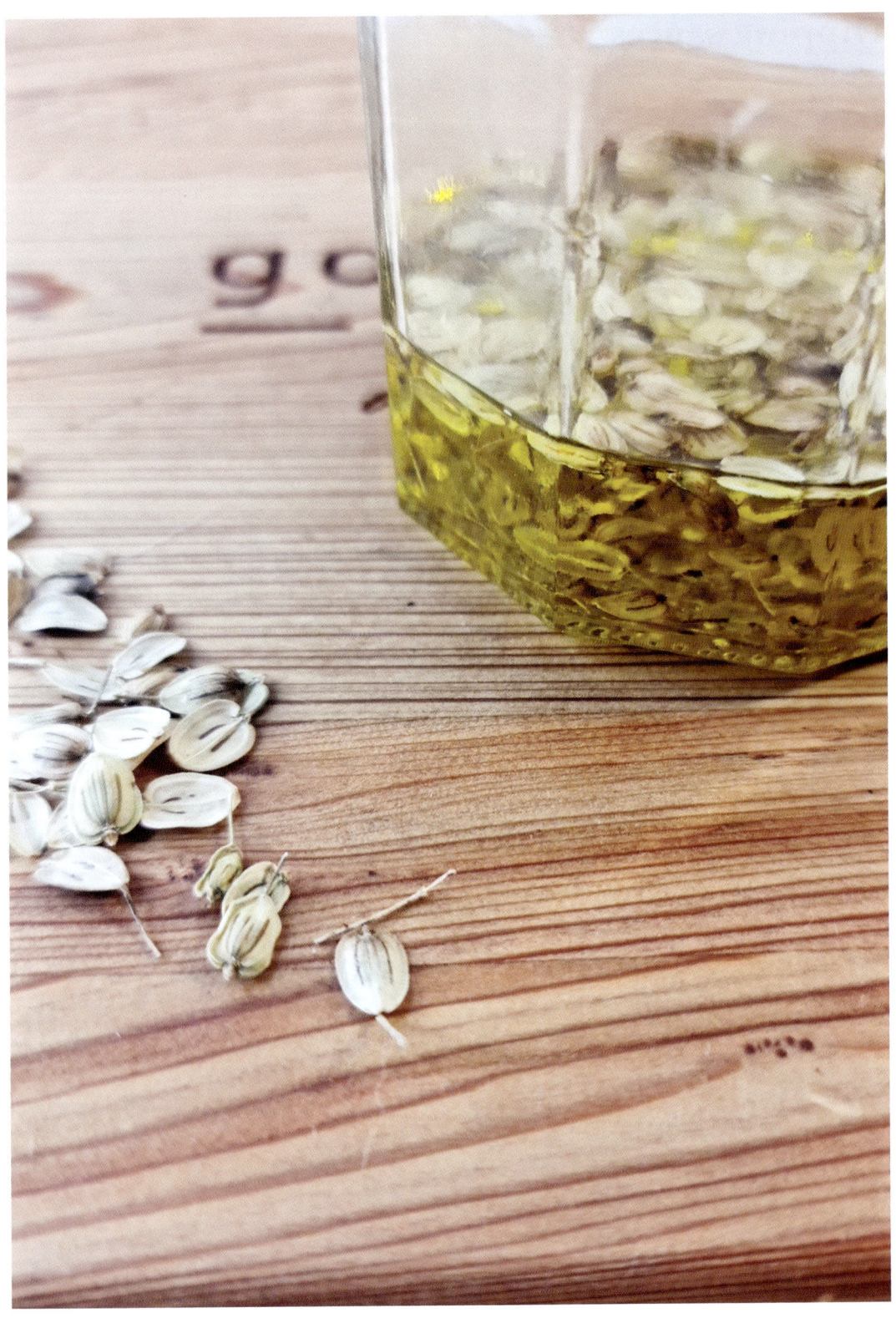

Hogweed seed dipping sauce

A pinch hogweed seed (they are particularly light seeds)
100ml olive oil

Add the olive oil to a sterilised jar.
Add in the hogweed seed.
Put the lid on the jar and gently shake so all of the seeds are coated in oil. Again, this is best a few days later as the oil takes on the flavour.

Foraged Condiments

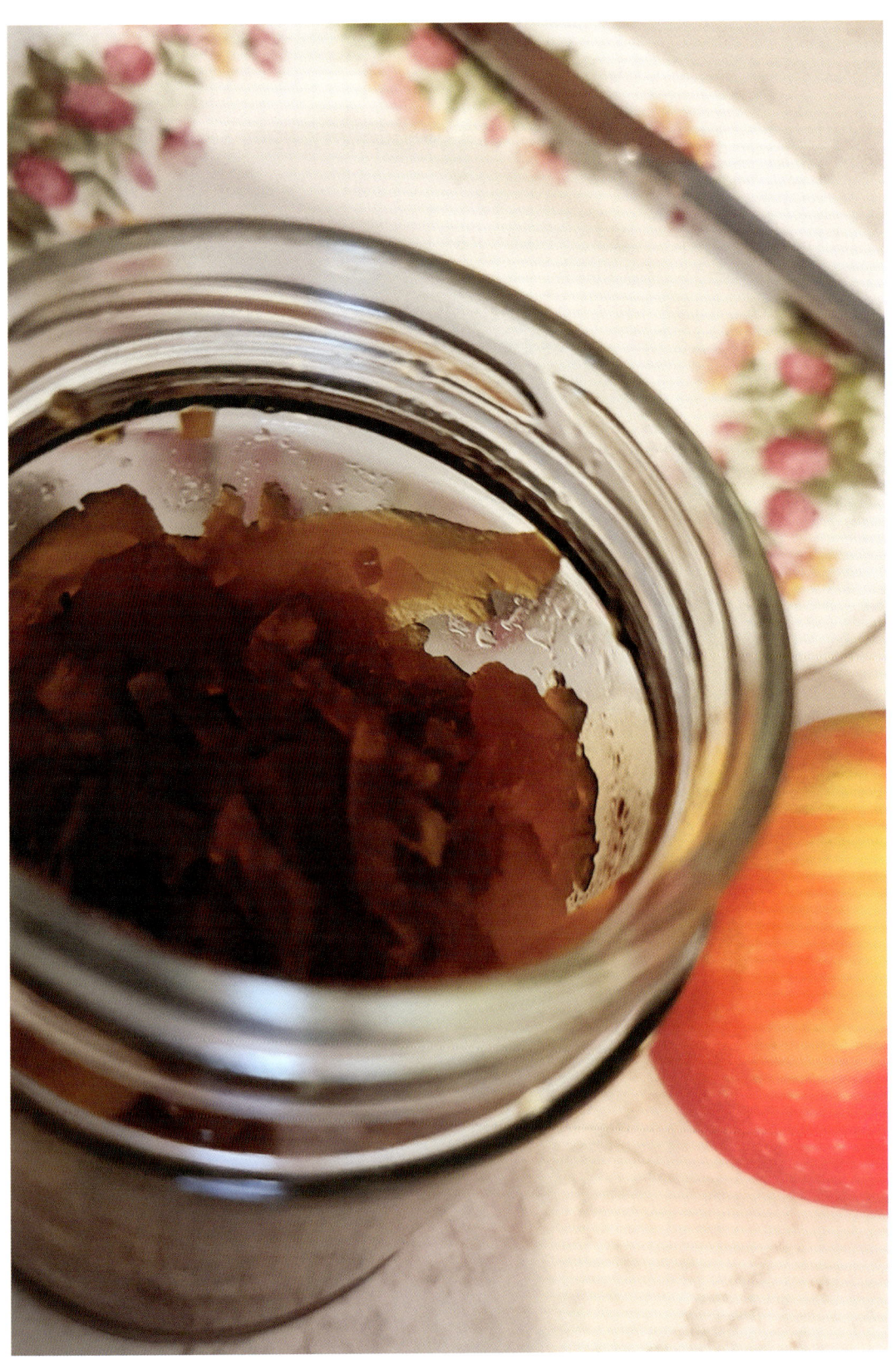

Chutneys

Apple and valerian flower chutney

For one small batch, which makes about two 300ml jars. Multiply for your requirements.

3 medium apples – chopped into about 1-inch cubes (I like leaving the skin on but if you want a smooth chutney, peel the apples. The skin will add texture if left on)
1 medium onion – chopped finely
3 heads valerian flowers, with flowers removed from the stalks
5 tablespoons vinegar
1 tablespoon oil
10g sugar
Salt to taste

Put the oil into a medium-sized saucepan. Use a medium heat and wait a few minutes. You want the onion to sizzle as it hits the pan. Add the onion to the heated oil and stir for a few minutes. Then add the chopped apple and allow to cook for about 5 minutes. Stir as required. Keep an eye on it. It's good to focus on the task in hand, and when we concentrate on one task that mind chatter should be focused.

Then add the vinegar and stir. Add the sugar and salt. This can be made with less sugar than the recipe says or have made it with no sugar as the sweetness of the apples is enough. But this is your chutney and it should be how you or its recipient wants it. That's one of the joys of making your own.

Continue to stir all the ingredients together, then add the valerian flowers. Keep stirring and eventually the apple will break down to give a saucy texture. This is when it is ready. Taste. It is about the balance of vinegar, sugars (including the apple) and salt. Adjust these to your liking.

Foraged Condiments

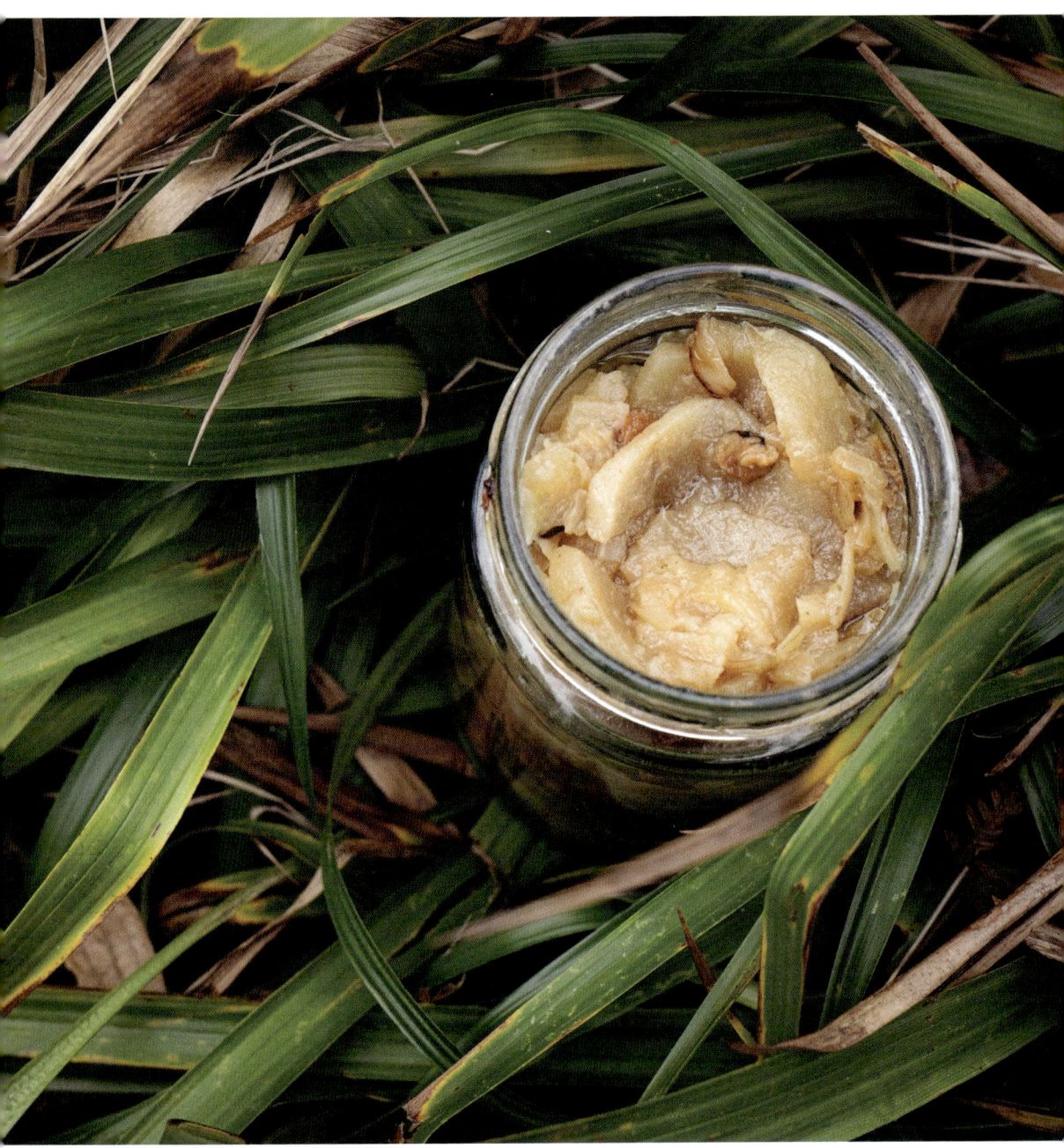

Pear and dandelion root chutney

3 medium pears, peeled and chopped into 2-inch pieces
1 onion, finely chopped
10g roasted dandelion root
7 tablespoons apple cider vinegar
10g sugar
1 tablespoon oil
Salt to taste

Put the oil into a medium-sized saucepan, set to a medium heat and wait a few minutes. You want the onion to sizzle as it hits the pan.

Add the onion to the heated oil and stir for a few minutes. Then add the chopped pears and allow to cook for about 5 minutes. Stir as required.

Then add the vinegar and stir. Then add the sugar and salt. This can be made with less sugar than the recipe says and or no sugar at all as the sweetness of the pears is enough.

Continue to stir all the ingredients together, then add the roasted dandelion roots. Keep stirring and eventually the pear will break down to give a saucy texture. Taste. Adjust the balance of vinegar, sugars and salt to your liking.

Foraged Condiments

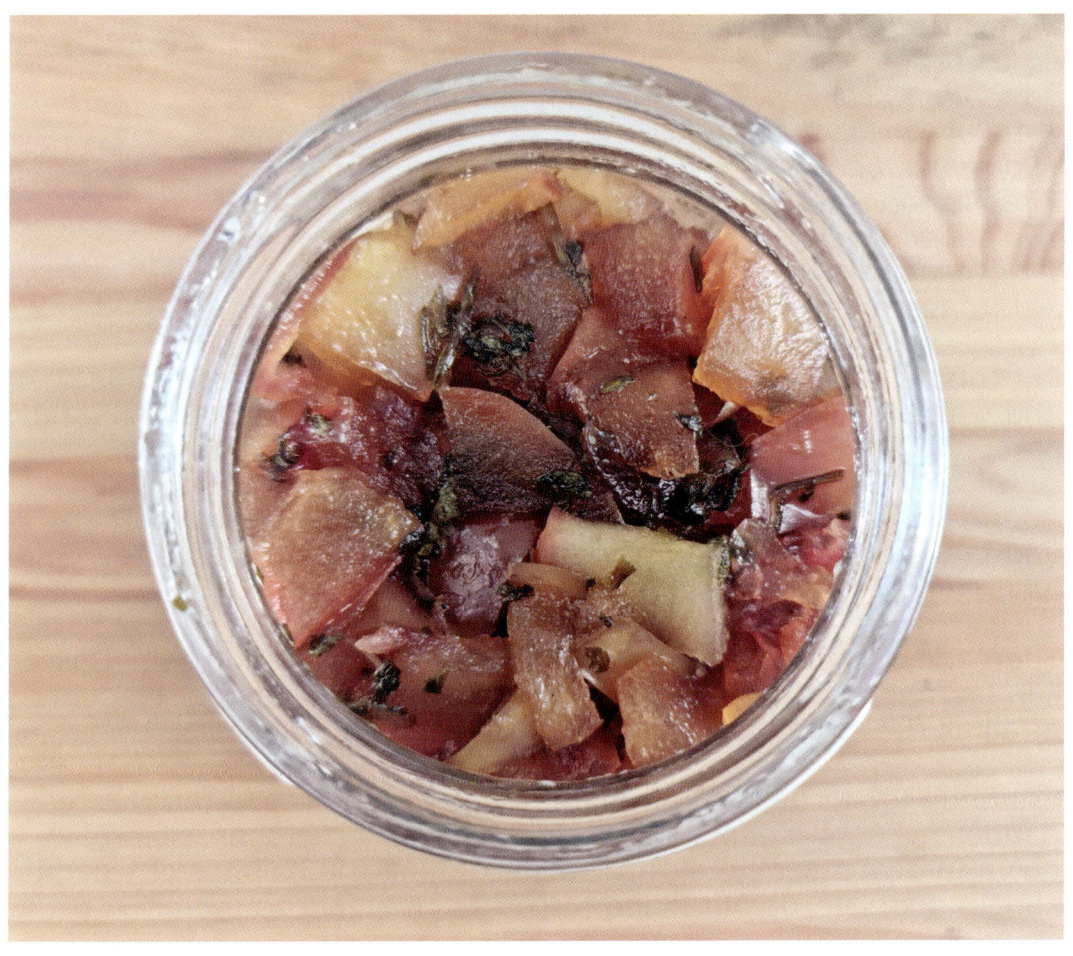

Sweet cicely and apple chutney

2 medium apples, chopped
3 sweet cicely flower heads, fresh and chopped
1 onion, finely chopped
100ml organic cider vinegar
10g sugar
1 tablespoon oil
Salt to taste

Heat up the oil in a medium pan and then add the chopped onion. Let it cook slowly until slightly brown, then add the apples and valerian flowers. Allow to cook for a few minutes then add the vinegar, sugar and salt. Let this cook until the apples start to break down, adding more vinegar if required.

Plantain leaf and bramble chutney

150g brambles
5 plantain leaves, chopped
1 small onion, finely chopped
100ml organic cider vinegar
5g sugar
Salt to taste

Heat up the oil in a medium pan and then add the chopped onion. Let it cook slowly until slightly brown, then add the brambles and plantain leaves. Allow these to cook for a few minutes, then add the vinegar, sugar and salt. Cook until the brambles start to break down, adding more vinegar if required.

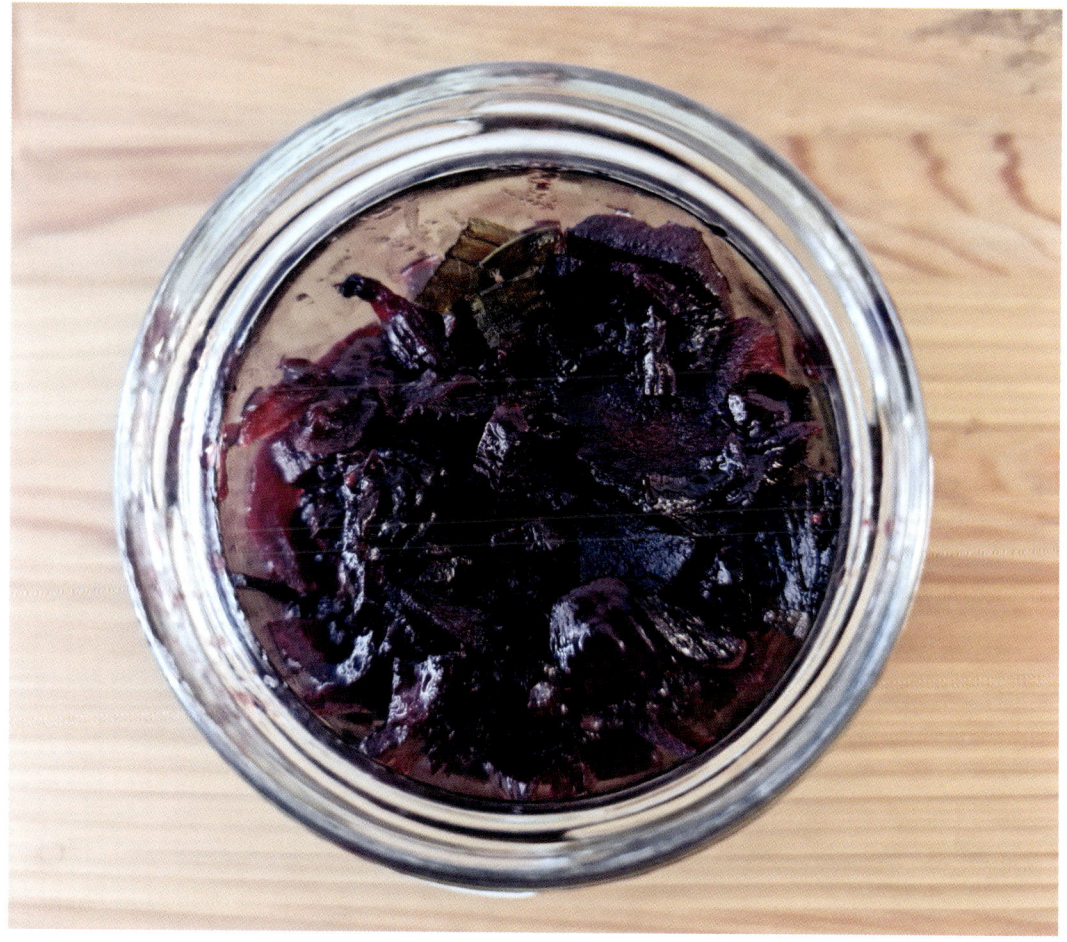

Foraged Condiments

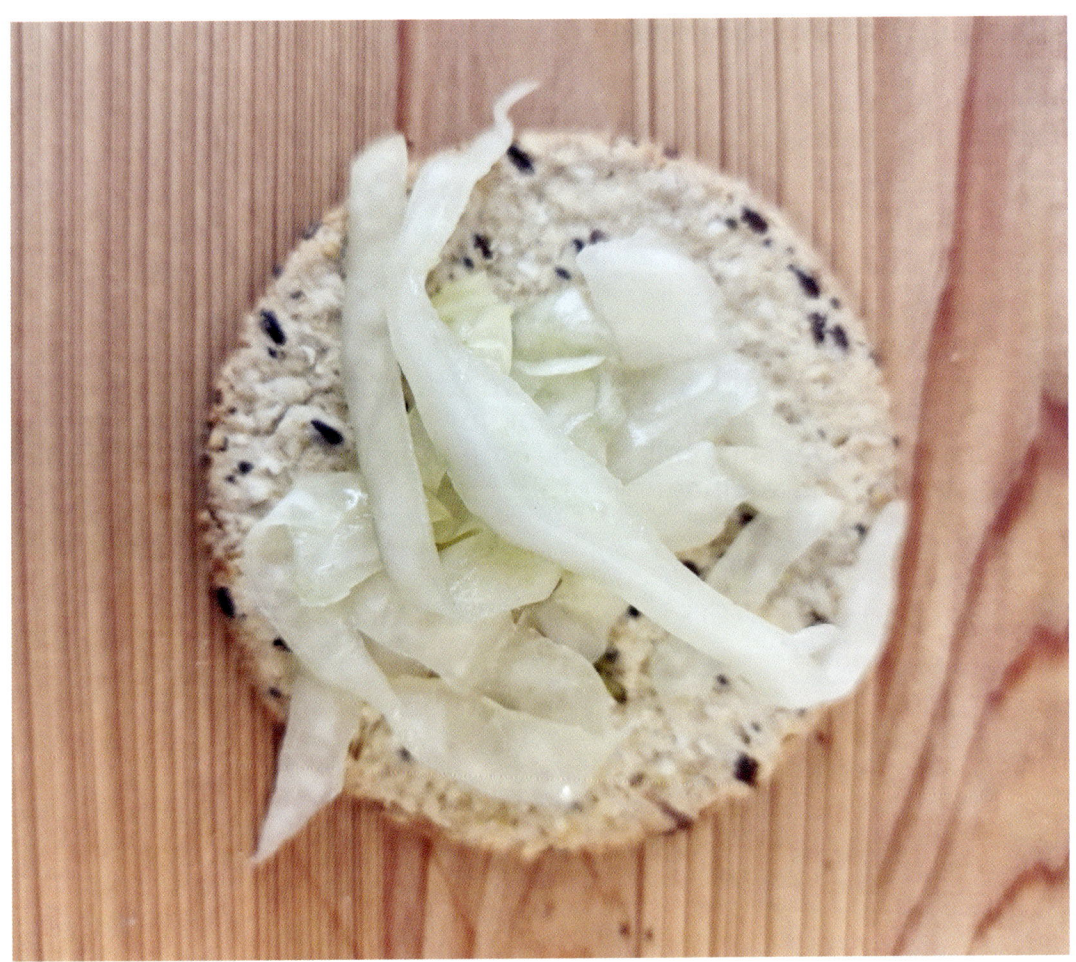

Ferments

There are whole books on the subject of fermentation, whether beer, wine, bread, cheese and a few others. It's a process folk have been doing for thousands of years for preserving food.

A very simple and basic ferment is the best one to start with. Fermentation needs no oxygen present so the healthy bacteria grow anaerobically, which means you need to keep everything below the water line.

Traditional cabbage sauerkraut

Prepare half a head of cabbage, white or red, and shred finely. Weigh your shredded cabbage and add 2–2.5% of sea salt. Work the salt into the cabbage with your hands.

Wait about 10 minutes. You will start to see some water at the bottom of the bowl the cabbage is in.

Then place this into clean, sterilised jars and add to water to top up.

You can buy fermenting stones to use as weights to keep the cabbage below the water or you can cut a cabbage leaf into shape and use a 'top'.

Seal, but not fully as the ferment will produce gases that need to be released.

Foraged Condiments

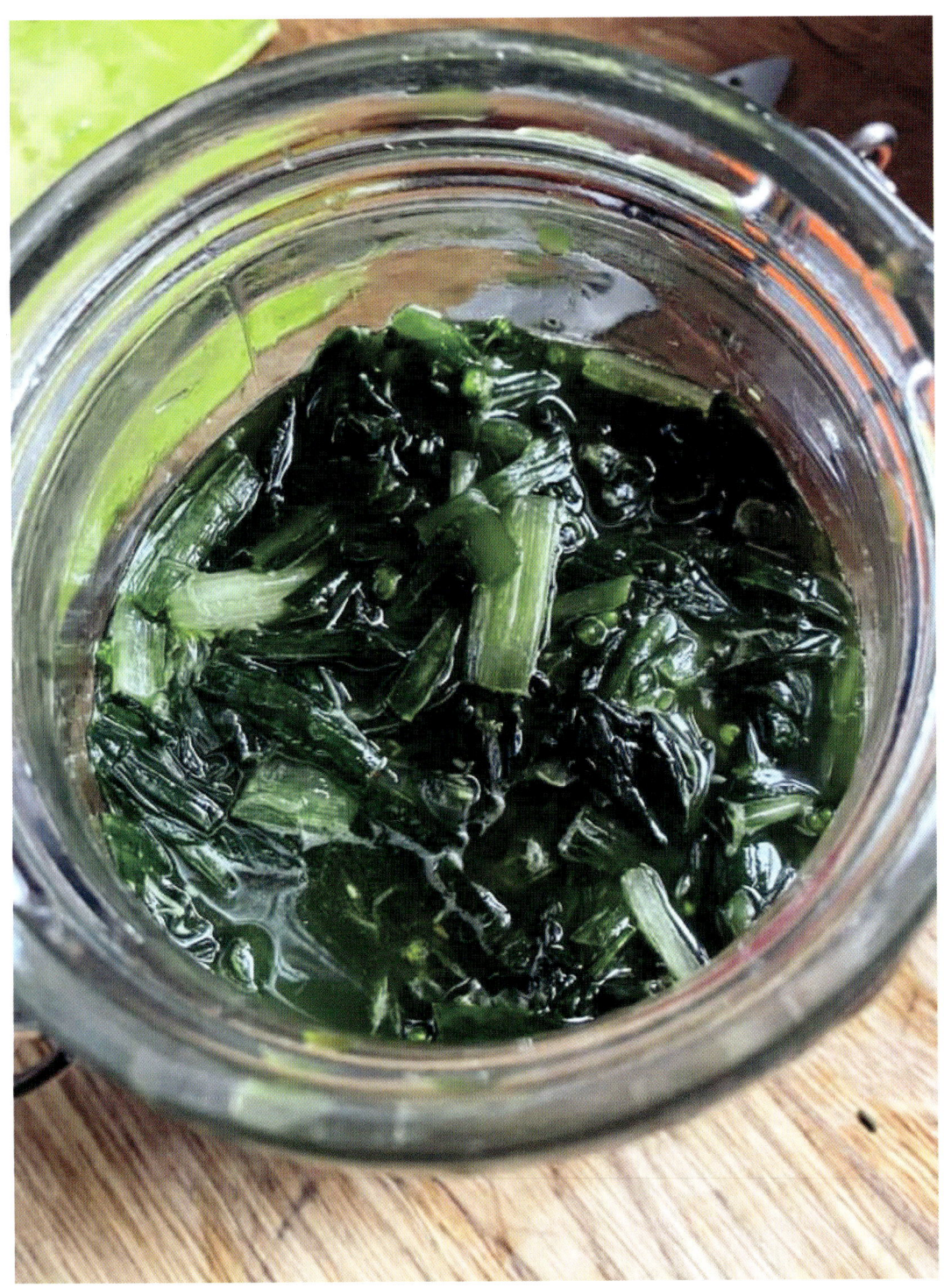

Fermented wild garlic

I love fermented wild garlic leaves, perhaps even more than the unfermented leaves.

Here a different technique can be used, which uses more equipment but is more fail-safe. Using a food vacuum packer, which means there is no way oxygen can get into the ferment as it is sealed.

Vacuum packer
Small to medium vacuum packer bags
Wild garlic leaves
Sea salt
Water

Weigh out the wild garlic leaves and add 2–2.5% of sea salt. I like 50g to a small vacuum bag. Or 100g to medium bag.

Then add water about a third of the way up the bag.

Place in the vacuum packer and seal accordingly. The time required will change from machine to machine.

Then label and put in a warm place: the ideal temperature is 25ºC.

Check every day and after about three days it is usually ready.

Open and taste and use if to your liking. If not, reseal and leave for a longer time.

Foraged Condiments

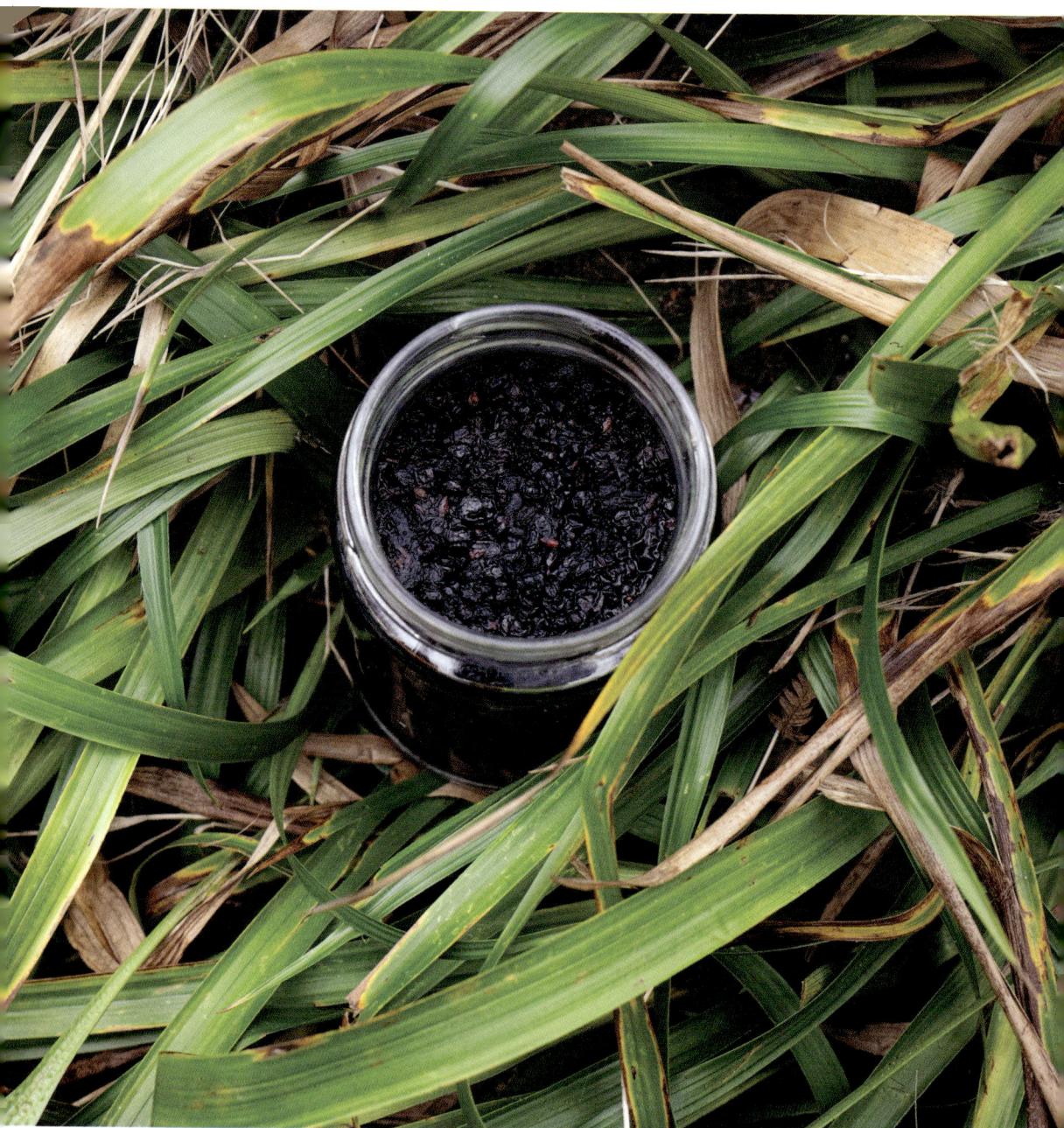

Jams and jellies

Elderberry jam

100g elderberries, taken off the stalks
1 apple for pectin
80g granulated sugar
Water

Place the fruit and the sugar into a pan and allow it to break down the fruit and dissolve the sugar. It will start to turn to a paste, and if too dry add some water, but not too much. The secret of jam is the temperature that it is taken to. You want it to reach between 103ºC and 106ºC. The sugar will allow you to reach above boiling point. It is worthwhile having a food thermometer to hand to test. Please be careful not to get the jam at this temperature on your skin.

Foraged Condiments

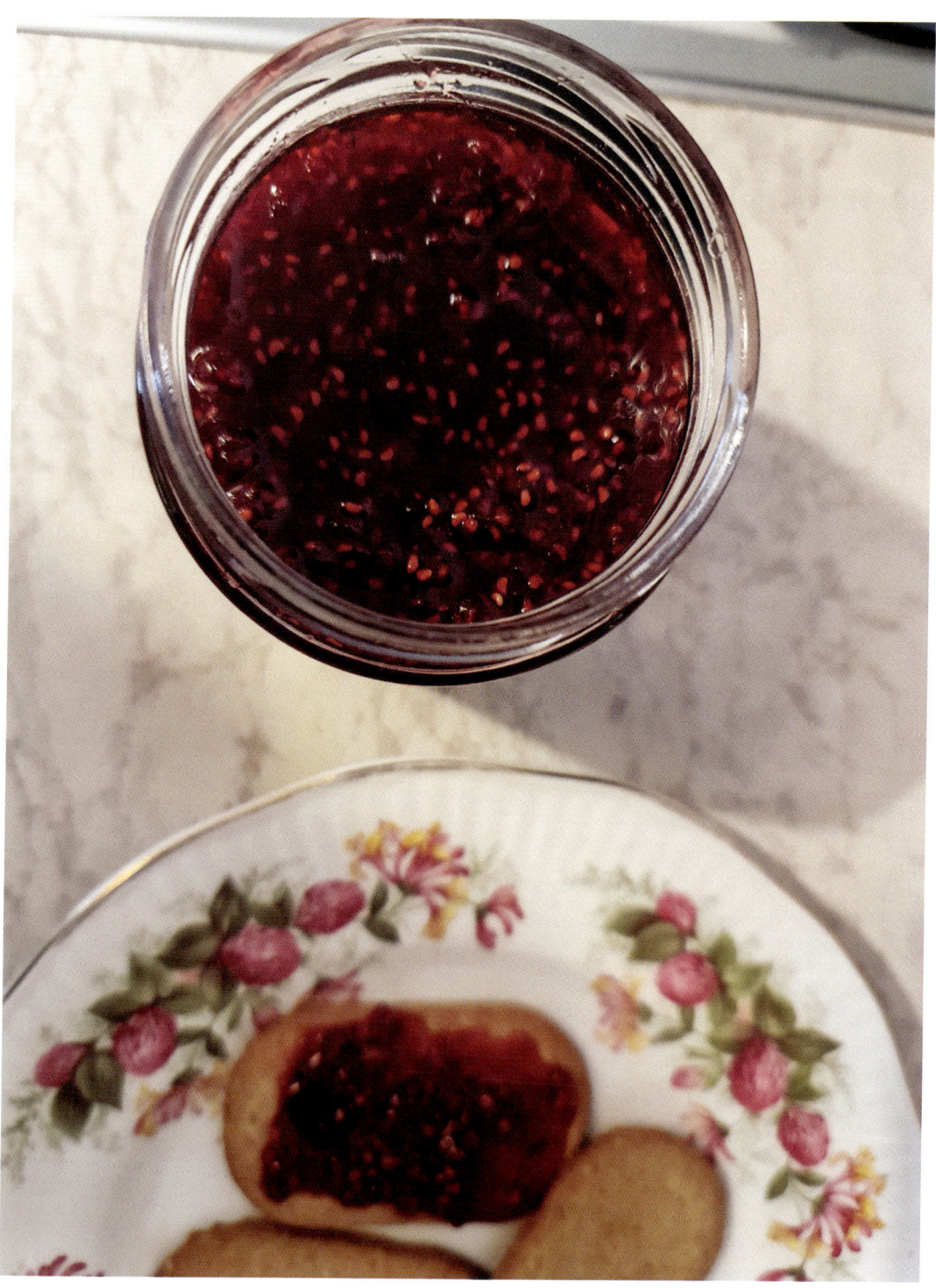

Wild raspberry jam

200g wild raspberries
1 apple, chopped into cubes
80g granulated sugar
Water

Place the fruit and the sugar into a pan and allow it to break down the fruit and dissolve the sugar. It will start to turn to a paste. If too dry, add some water, but not too much.

The secret of jam is the temperature that it is taken to. You want it to reach between 103ºC and 106ºC. The sugar will allow you to reach above boiling point. It is worthwhile having a food thermometer to hand to test. Please be careful not to get the jam at this temperature on your skin.

Foraged Condiments

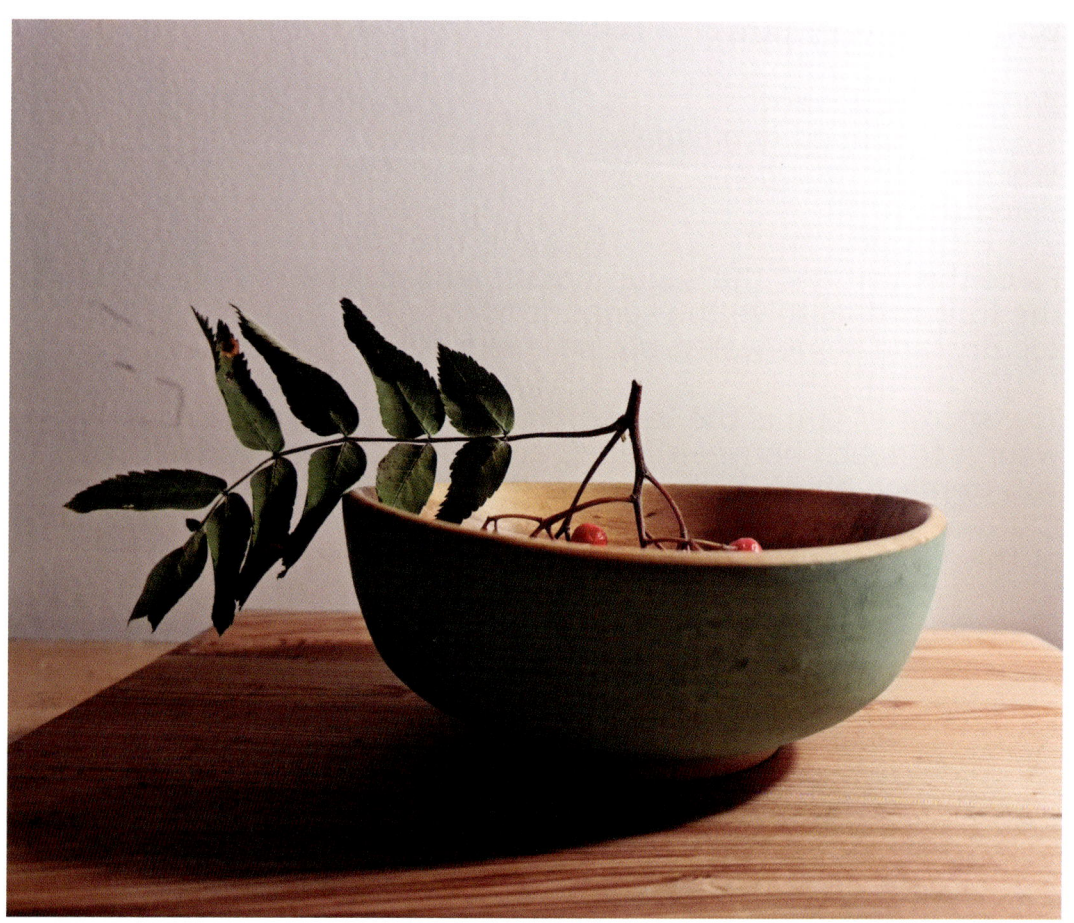

Rowan berry jelly

250g rowan berries
150g granulated sugar
Water

Boil the fruit and strain by allowing the juice to drip through a jelly bag or muslin cloth overnight.

Place the fruit juice and the sugar into a pan and heat to dissolve the sugar. The secret of jelly is the temperature that it is taken to. You want it to reach between 103ºC and 106ºC. The sugar will allow you to reach above boiling point. It is worthwhile having a food thermometer to hand to test. Please be careful not to get the jelly at this temperature on your skin.

Foraged Condiments

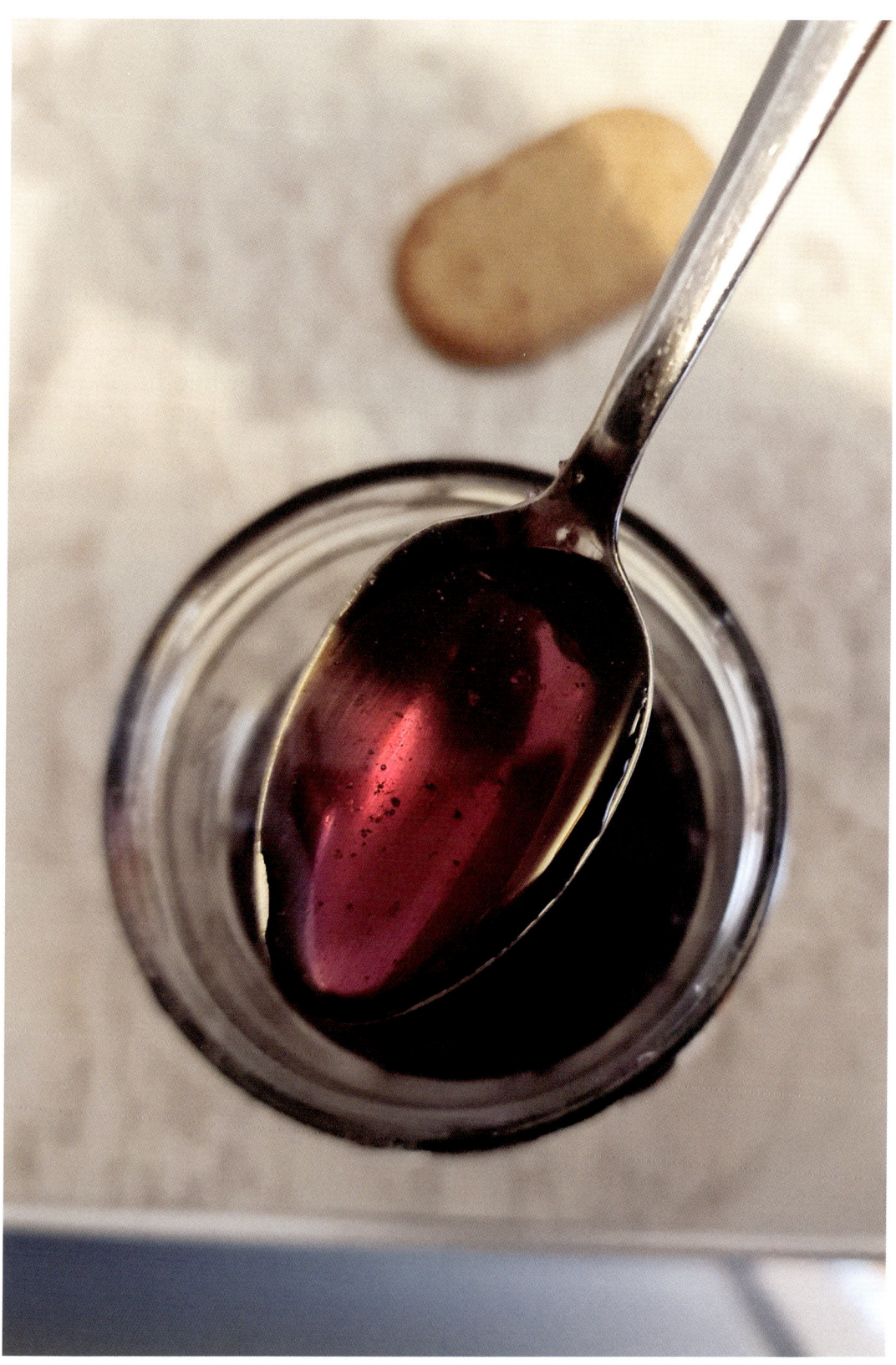

Rosebay willowherb flower jam

100g rosebay willowherb flowers
1 apple, chopped into cubes
80g granulated sugar
Water

Place the fruit, flowers and the sugar into a pan and allow it to break down the fruit and dissolve the sugar and start to turn to a paste. If too dry, add some water, but not too much.

The secret of jam is the temperature that it is taken to. You want it to reach between 103ºC and 106ºC. The sugar will allow you to reach above boiling point. It is worthwhile having a food thermometer to hand to test. Please be careful not to get the jam at this temperature on your skin.

Foraged Condiments

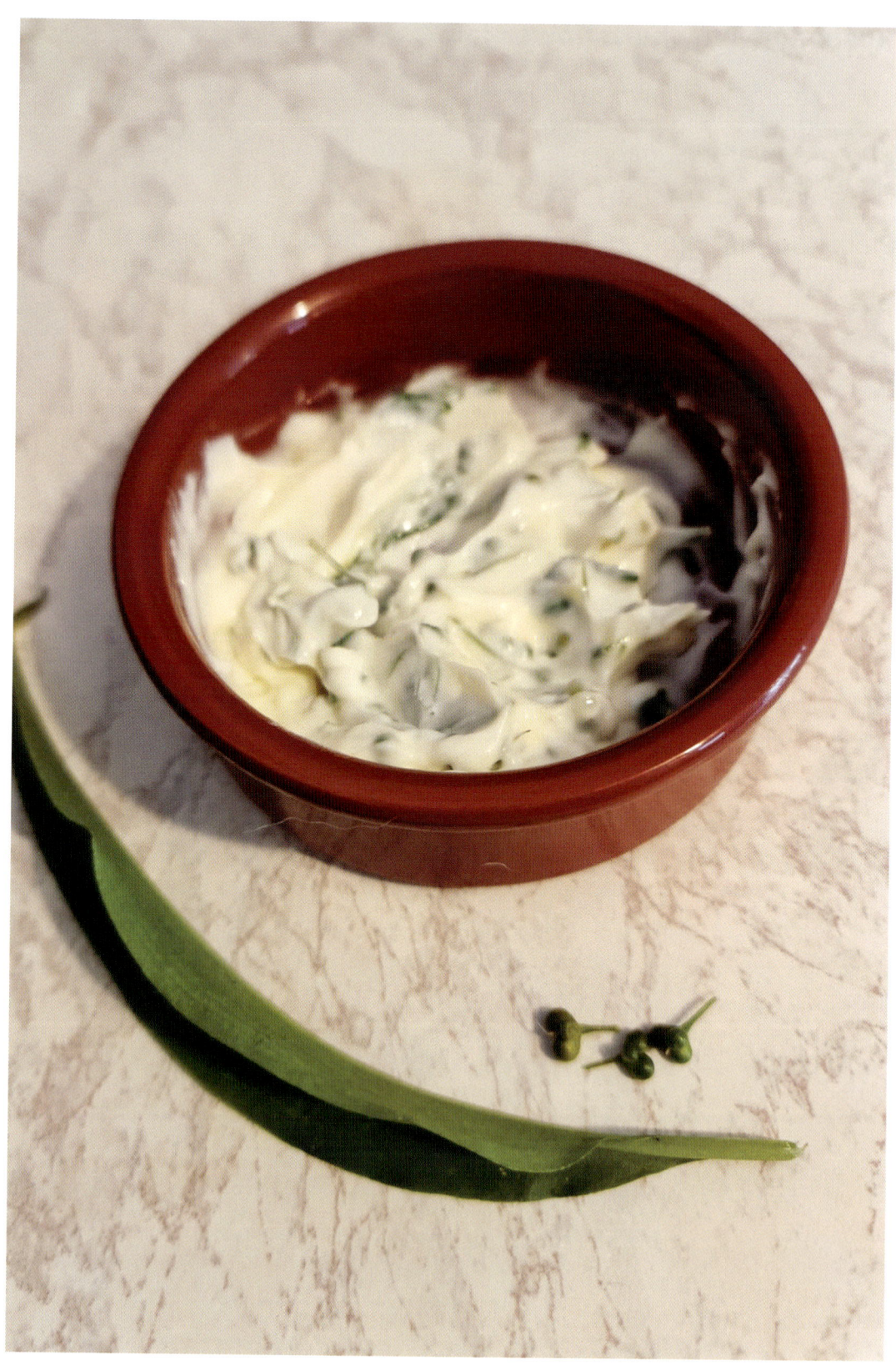

Aiolis and pestos

Wild garlic bud aioli

5 wild garlic flower buds
50g mayonnaise
Sea salt to taste

Mash up the wild garlic buds lightly, add with the salt to mayonnaise and mix.

Jack by the hedge aioli

3 medium Jack by the hedge leaves, finely shredded
50g mayonnaise
Sea salt

Take the finely shredded Jack by the hedge leaves and salt, add to mayonnaise and mix.

Foraged Condiments

Spring pesto

8 nettle tops
A handful young cleavers tops
A handful wild garlic leaves
15 young ground elder leaves
10 dandelion young leaves before flowering
150ml olive oil
50g nuts hazelnuts/cashews/almonds/pine nuts
Juice half a lemon
Sea salt

Put everything in a blender and mash it all together. Add more oil if dry, and add more leaves and nuts if too loose. You are looking for the consistency of a paste. This is a delicious pesto that can be used traditionally to add to pasta or anyway you like.

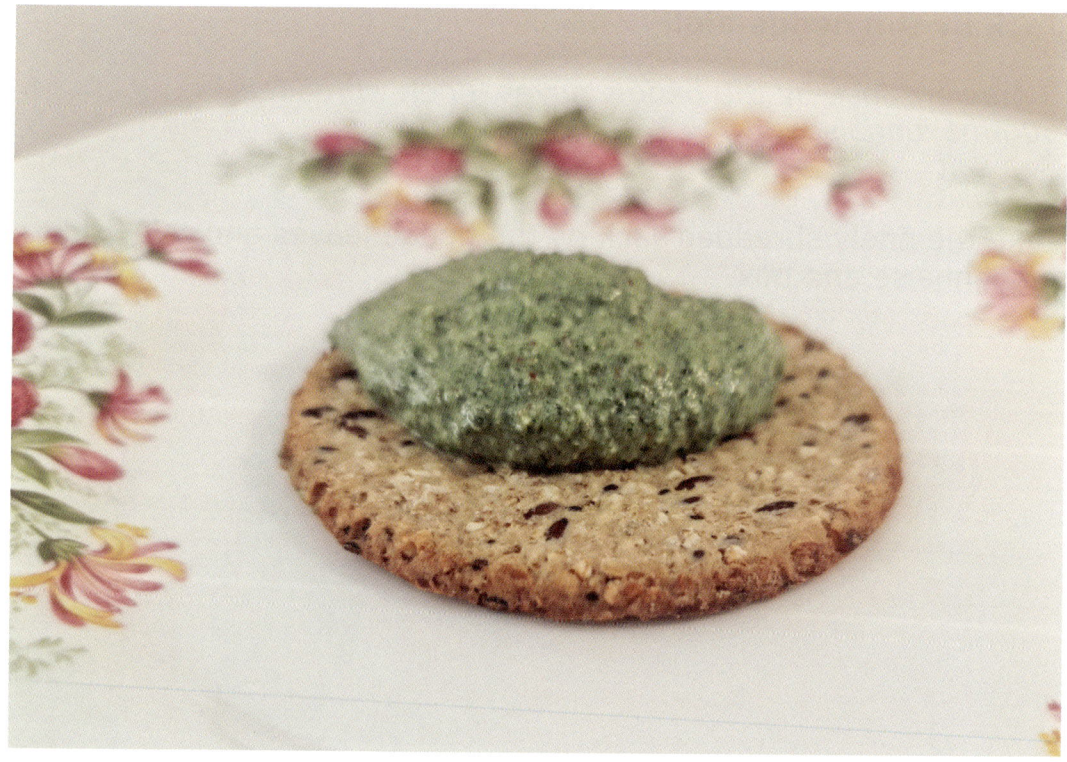

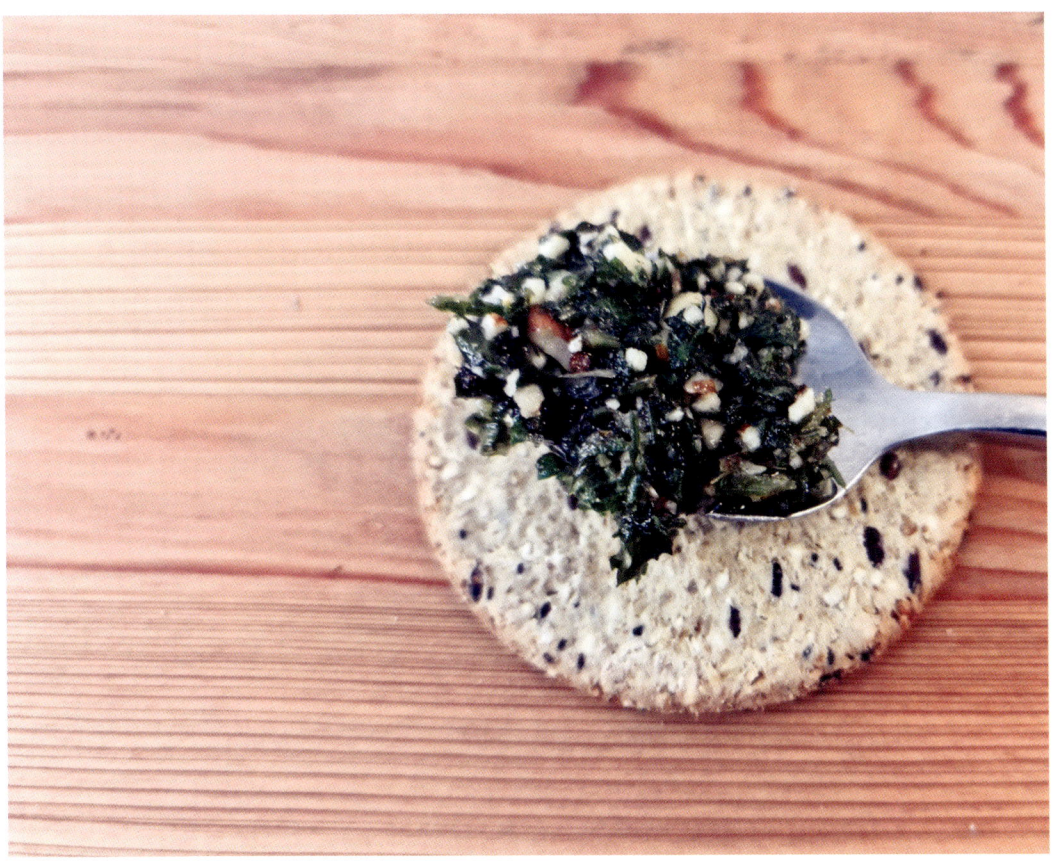

Nettle and hazelnut pesto

A handful young nettle leaves
30g hazelnuts
Juice half of lemon
100ml olive oil
3 cloves garlic, crushed
Sea salt to taste

Add all the ingredients into a blender and blend into a paste texture. Add more oil if too dry and more nuts or nettle leaves if too moist. Make it as you want it, playing with the salt, lemon juice and garlic to perfect it to your taste.

Wild garlic pesto

A handful of wild garlic leaves
100ml olive oil
Half juice of a lemon
Nuts of your choice (hazelnuts are my favourite, cashews make it creamier)
Sea salt

Add all the ingredients to a blender and blend for a short time. If too dry add more oil, if too moist add more nuts and leaves. The traditional way of making pesto is by mortar and pestle, but this takes more time and more arm strength. All the same it is a lovely process of watching it all come together.

Salad dressings

Olive oil and fermenting juice salad dressing

50ml olive oil
50ml ferment juice from a sauerkraut
1 clove garlic, crushed
Sea salt
Black pepper

This is very simple salad dressing that gives a great punch of flavour to the salad. Add all the ingredients to a mug or jar, and whisk with a fork until it becomes creamy. Pour over your salad.

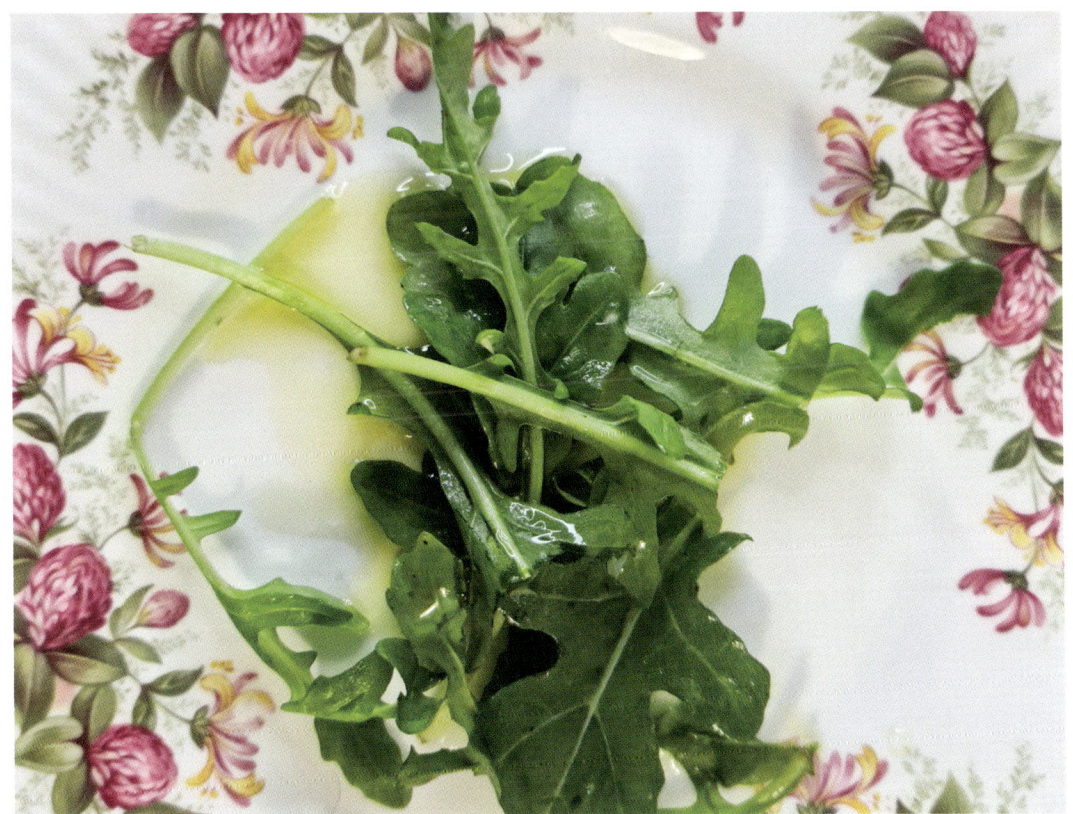

Wild garlic and elderberry vinegar dressing

30ml wild garlic infused oil
20ml elderberry vinegar
Sea salt

Another simple salad dressing. Place all the ingredients into a mug or jar and whisk with a fork until it is starts to look creamy. Pour over your salad.

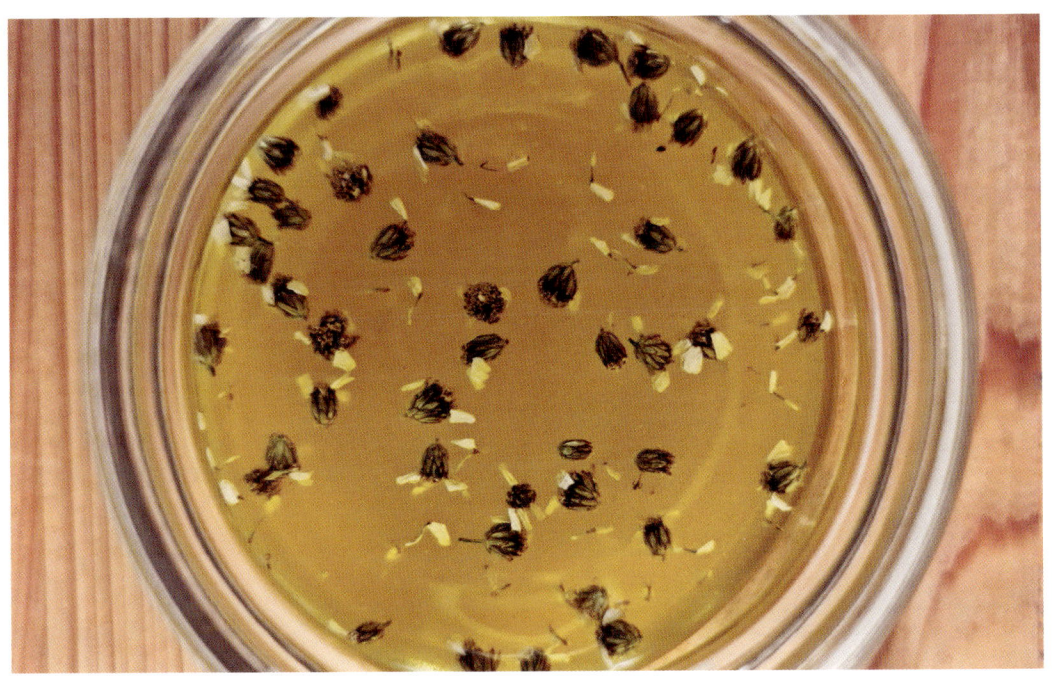

Yarrow flower salad dressing

30ml olive oil
Juice of half a lemon
1 flower head of yarrow, with the small flowers removed
1 dollop of honey, quarter of teaspoon
Salt to taste

Add all of the ingredients into a mug or jar and whisk with a fork until it starts to look creamy, then pour over your chosen salad.

Foraged Condiments

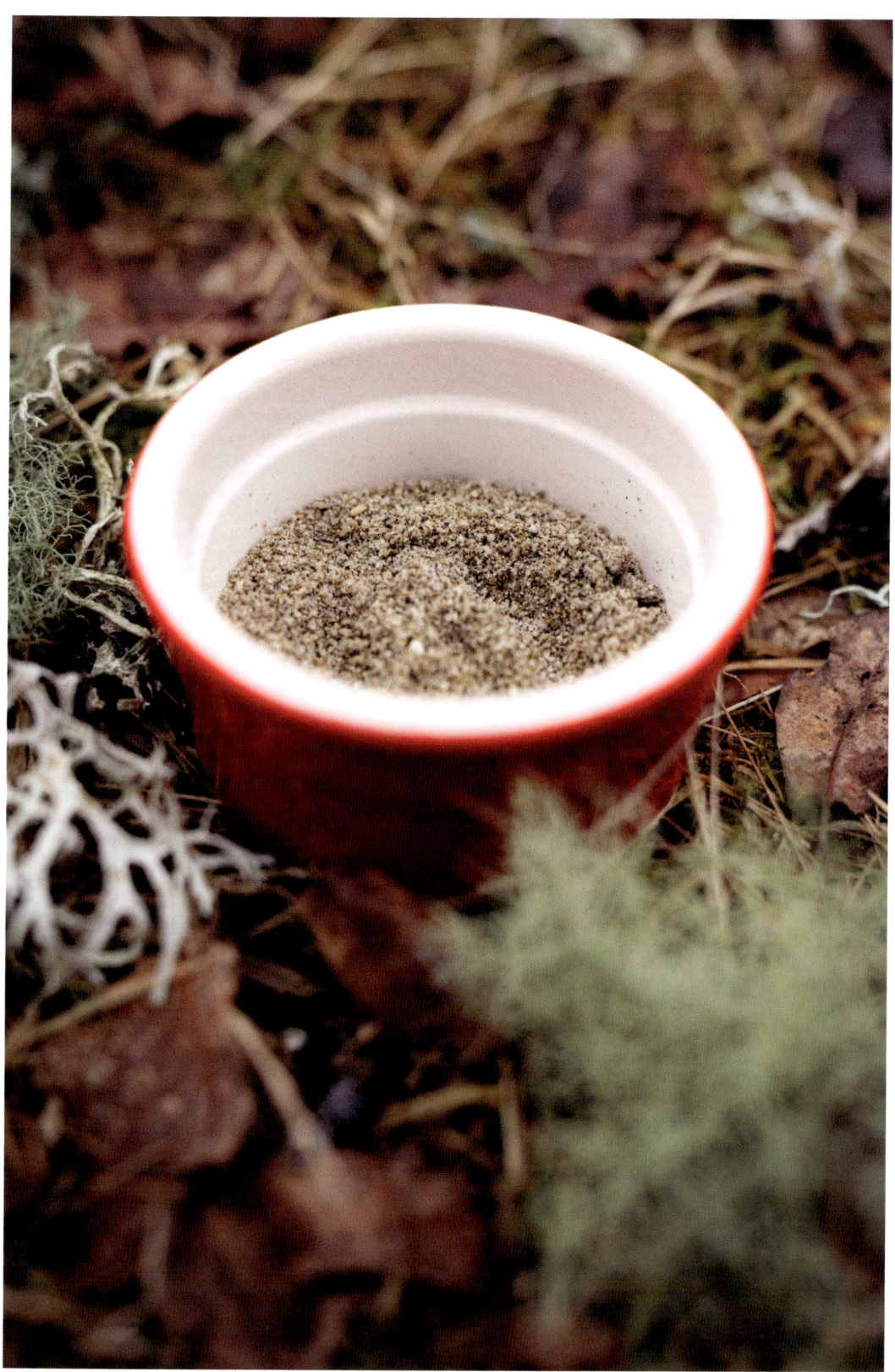

Salts and a sugar

Nettle seed gomasio

30g nettle seed
60g sesame seed
10g sea salt

Put the salt in a blender and powder it. Then remove it and powder the nettle seed and sesame together. Add the salt back in and blend for a very short time. This is delicious over eggs.

Foraged Condiments

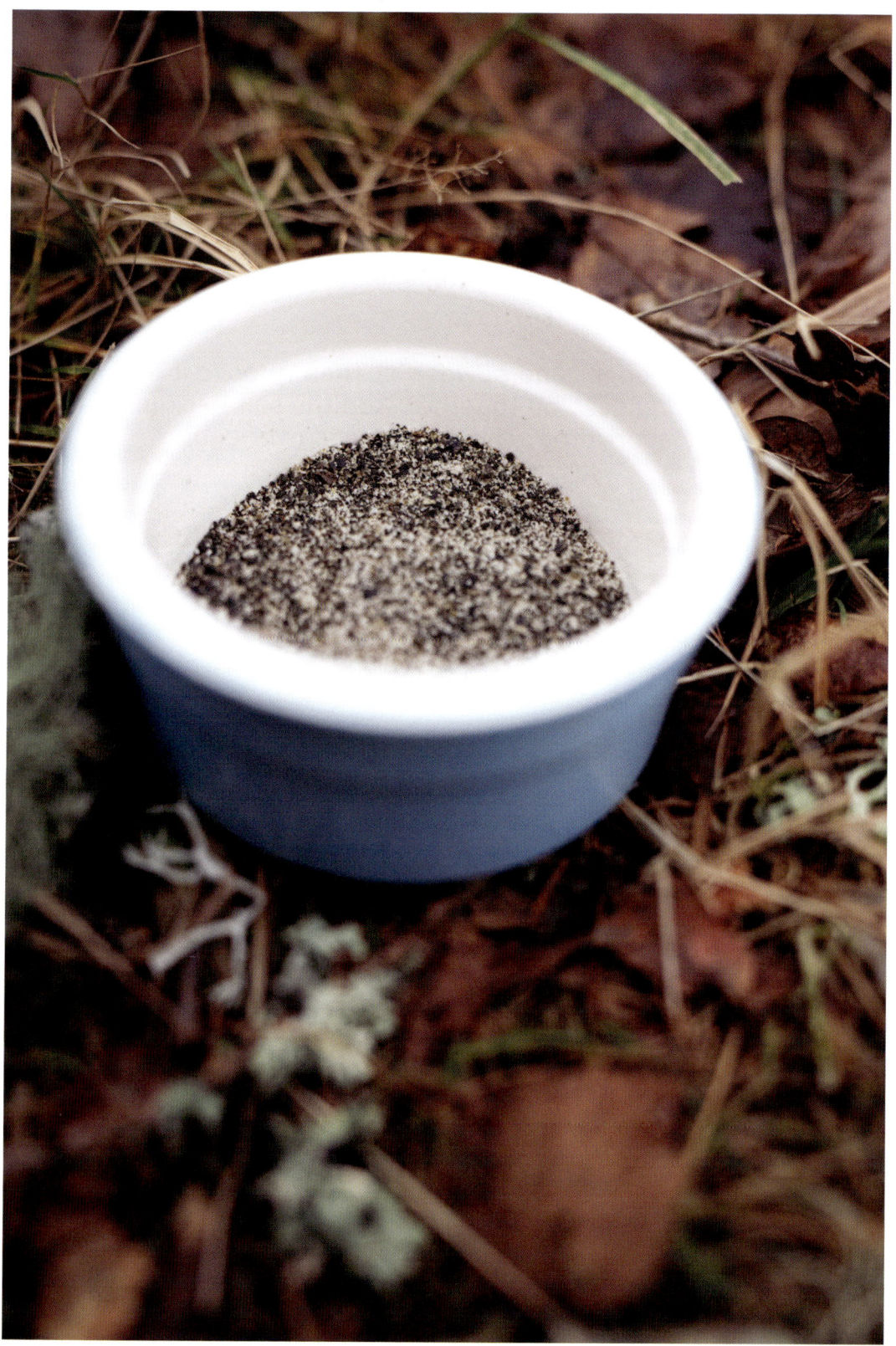

Seaweed salt

30g dried pepper dulse (peppery) or sugar kelp (sweeter)
10g sea salt

First blend the salt into a powder, then add the dried seaweed. Blend for a short time. Store in an airtight container.

Plantain seed salt

25g plantain seeds (when young will taste of mushrooms and when slightly older will taste nutty)
10g sea salt
20g hazelnuts

First place in the salt into your blender and whizz it up to make it more powdery. Then add the plantain seeds and hazelnuts, and give it a short blast. Store in an airtight container.

Foraged Condiments

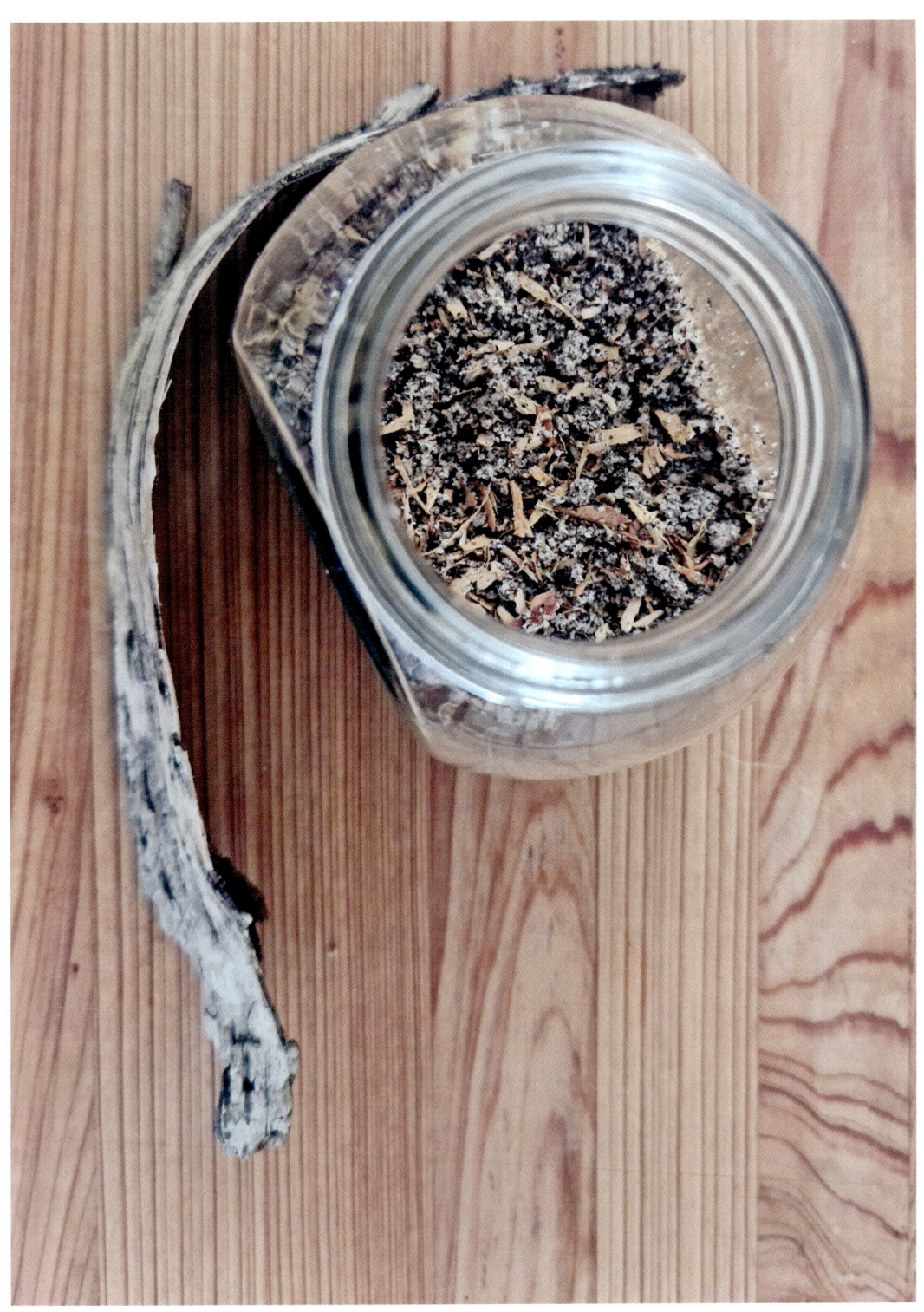

Birch bark salt

10g birch bark or a small piece, dried
25g hazelnuts
5g salt

Add all the ingredients into a blender, blast for a while and remove. Place in an airtight container.

Foraged Condiments

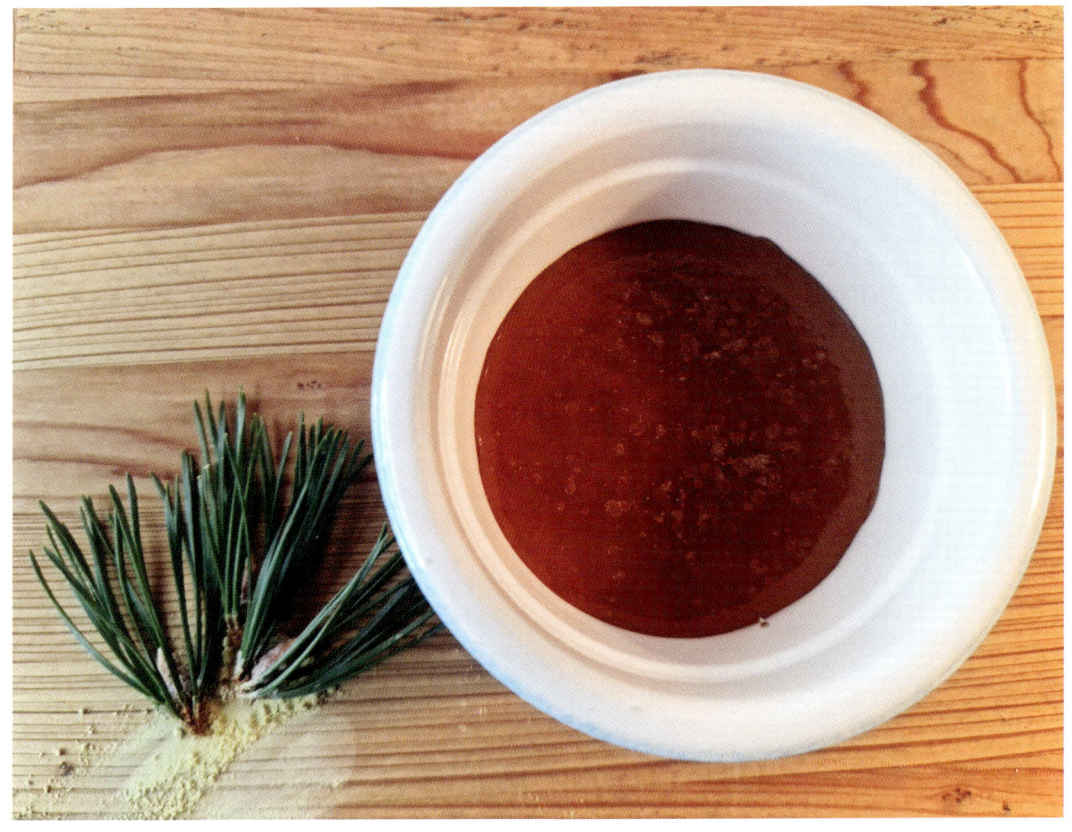

Pine pollen sugar

250ml water
250g sugar
5g pine pollen

Heat the water and sugar together in a saucepan until it reaches 115ºC and 118ºC, then remove from the boil. Be very careful as this mixture can burn easily. On slight cooling add the pine pollen and stir well. Pour into a container that will allow the mixture to be the shape you want it to be when set. Allow to set overnight. You can score the mixture to give easier breaking once set.

Ketchups

Hawthorn ketchup

100g hawthorn berries, destoned
1 onion
1 apple
5 tomatoes
30ml apple cider vinegar
10g sugar or to taste
5g sea salt or to taste
15ml oil, preferably sunflower oil

Chop the onion, tomatoes and apple into small chunks. Put the oil in a pan and turn to a medium heat. Add the chopped onion and allow it cook until translucent, stirring from time to time so it doesn't brown.

Then add the apple and tomatoes, sugar, salt and vinegar. Stir well and keep stirring for a few minutes. Then add the destoned hawthorn berries – a fiddly job and best done beforehand. Cook for as long as the ingredients are all cooked through and start to create a chunky sauce. Remove from the heat and allow to cool. Then blitz it with a hand blender or into a blender. Put into sterilised jars or sauce bottle and keep in the fridge.

Rosehip ketchup

100g dried rosehips or 50g of fresh rosehip hulls. (Remove the seeds and all the hairs – don't leave any hairs as they are an irritant. I find muslin cloth does the job well, but I triple up the cloth.)
1 medium onion, chopped into chunks
1 medium apple or pear, chopped into chunks
30ml apple cider vinegar
10g sugar or to taste
5g salt or to taste
15ml oil, preferably sunflower oil

Add the oil to a pan and turn to a medium heat. Allow the oil to heat up, then add the onion. Cook it gently for a few minutes until it is translucent, then add the apple or pear. Stir and cook for a few more minutes. Add the sugar, salt and vinegar, then the rosehips.

Allow this to cook until the apple or pear gets soft and the rosehips break down. This will take longer if using dried rosehips. Add a bit water if needs be to stop it sticking to the bottom of the pan. Take off the heat and allow to cool.

Then using either an handheld blender or a countertop one make the sauce smooth. Transfer into a sterilised jar or sauce bottle. Keep in the fridge.

Sauces, stuffings and a coating

Hawthorn spiced sauce

100g hawthorn berries, destoned
50ml apple cider vinegar
25g sugar
5g salt
1 clove garlic, mashed
1 tablespoon of five-spice powder

Cook the hawthorn berries in some water until they are mushy. Strain them through some muslin cloth, then return the liquid to the pan. Then add the vinegar, sugar, salt, garlic and five-spice powder. Cook until it reduces down into a thick paste.

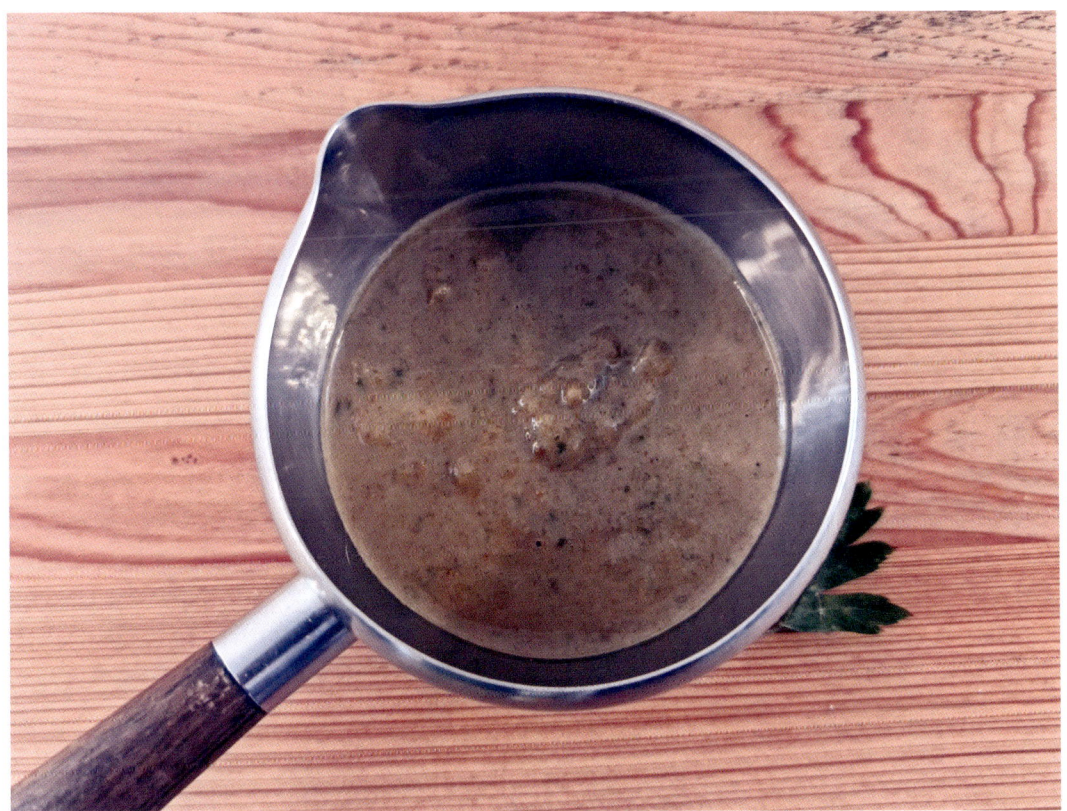

Beetroot and hogweed seed sauce

3 roasted beetroots
1 onion, chopped in chunks
3g hogweed seed
50ml apple cider vinegar
10g sugar
3g sea salt
15ml oil, preferably sunflower oil

Add the oil to a pan and put on a medium heat. Allow the oil to heat up, then add the onion. Cook it gently for a few minutes until it is translucent then add the beetroots. Stir and cook for a few more minutes. Add the sugar, salt and vinegar, then add the hogweed seeds. Allow this to cook until the beetroots get soft. Add a little water, if needs be, to stop it sticking to the bottom of the pan. Take off the heat and allow to cool. Then, using either a handheld blender or a counter top one, make the sauce smooth. Transfer into a sterilised jar or sauce bottle. Keep in the fridge.

Ground elder cooking paste

1 onion, chopped finely
5 leaves ground elder, using young leaves before flowering
1 teaspoon sugar
Half a teaspoon salt
1 tablespoon oil

Heat the oil up in a pan. Add the finely chopped onion and allow to cook until translucent. Then add the sugar and salt, and reduce the heat. The onions will eventually caramelise and turn a light brown colour. Then add the chopped ground elder and slowly mix together. Once the ground elder is wilted and incorporated remove from the heat.

This can be used as a basis for many recipes.

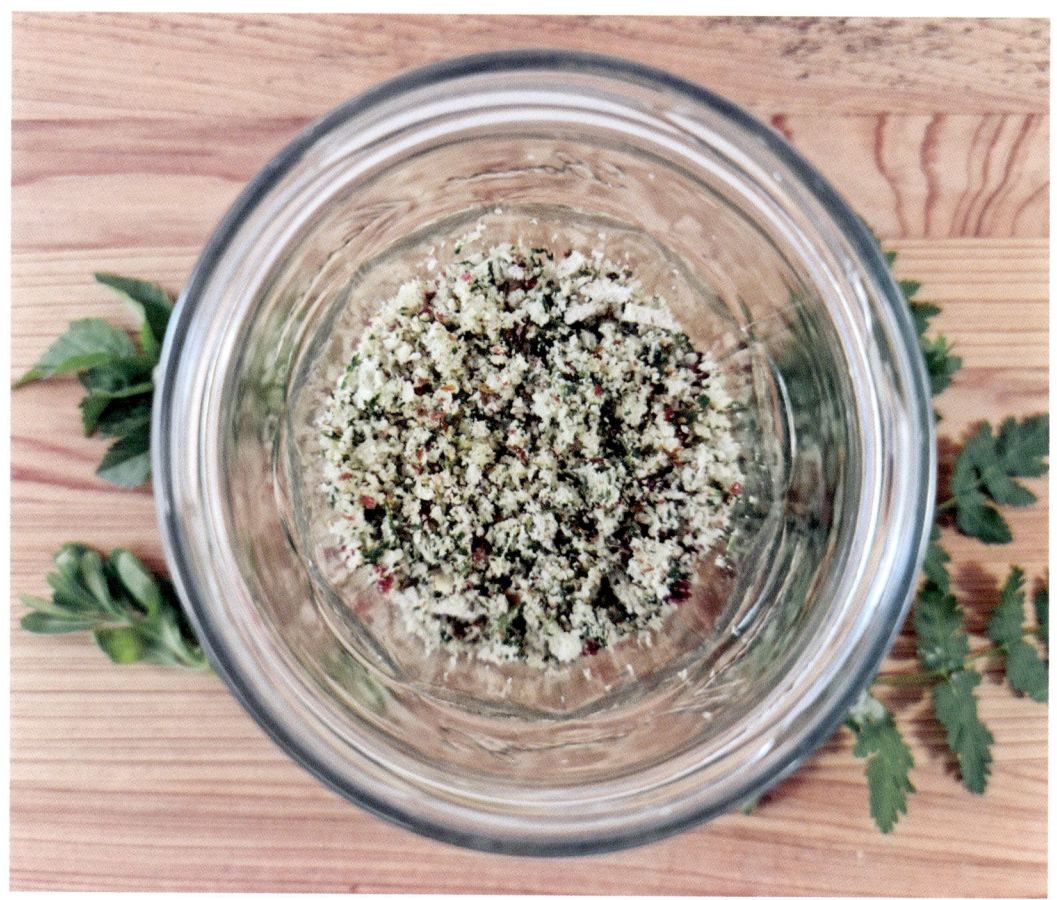

Wild stuffing mix

5 nettle tops
3 ground elder leaves
1 sprig young cleavers
50g breadcrumbs

Put all the ingredients into a blender and whizz up.

Use as you would any stuffing mix.

Foraged Condiments

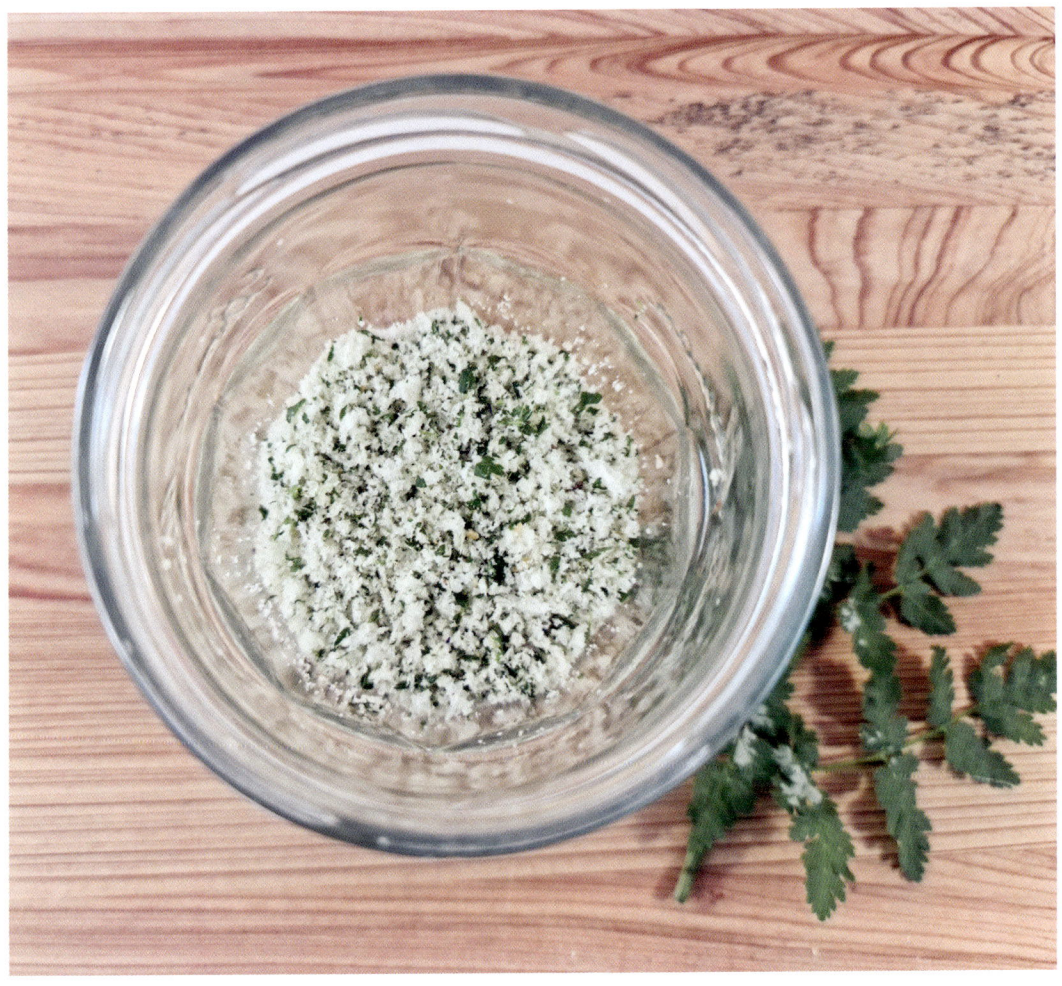

Sweet cicely coating

5 sprigs sweet cicely leaves
50g breadcrumbs

Put both ingredients in a blender and whizz up. This coating is particularly good with fish.

Vinegars

Elderberry vinegar

100g elderberries
150g sugar
250ml apple cider vinegar

Flavoured vinegars are very easy to make. You steep the elderberries in the vinegar – just therberries, and no stalks. I prefer to do this over a day or two, then drain therberries from the vinegar and place this vinegar into a pan. Gently heat, then add the sugar until it dissolves. Allow to cool, then add to a sterilised jar or vinegar bottle.

Bramble vinegar

100g brambles
150g sugar
250ml apple cider vinegar

Steep the brambles in the vinegar. I prefer to do this over a day or two, then drain the brambles from the vinegar and place the vinegar in a pan. Gently heat, then add the sugar until it dissolves. Allow to cool, then add to a sterilised jar or vinegar bottle.

Foraged Condiments

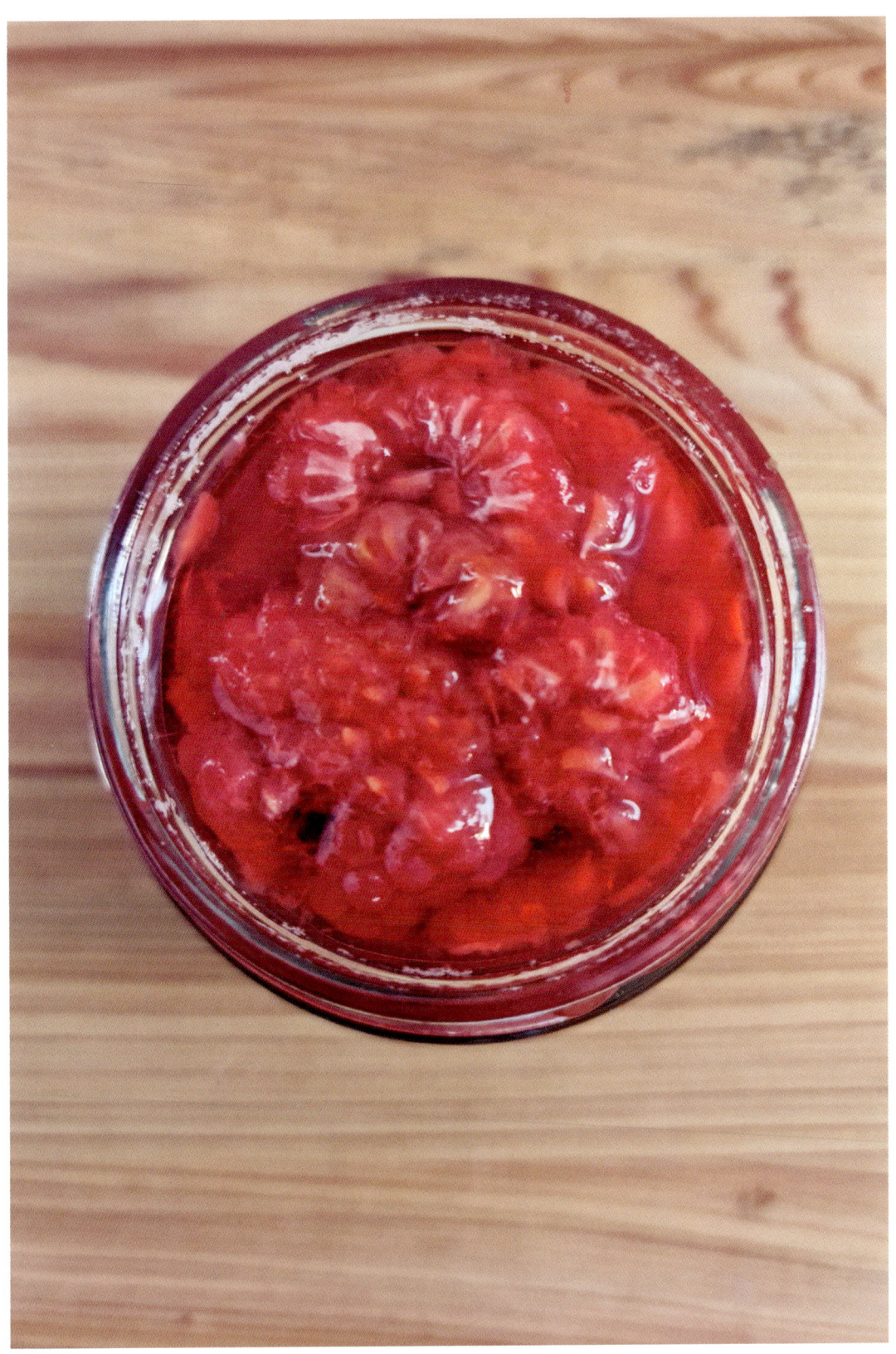

Pickles

Pickled wild raspberries

100g wild raspberries
80ml cider vinegar
10g sugar
5g salt

Put the raspberries and vinegar into a pan, heating gently until the raspberries break down. Then add the sugar and salt. Let the sugar and salt dissolve, then allow the mixture to cool and place into a sterilised jar. Don't put the lid on until it has fully cooled down.

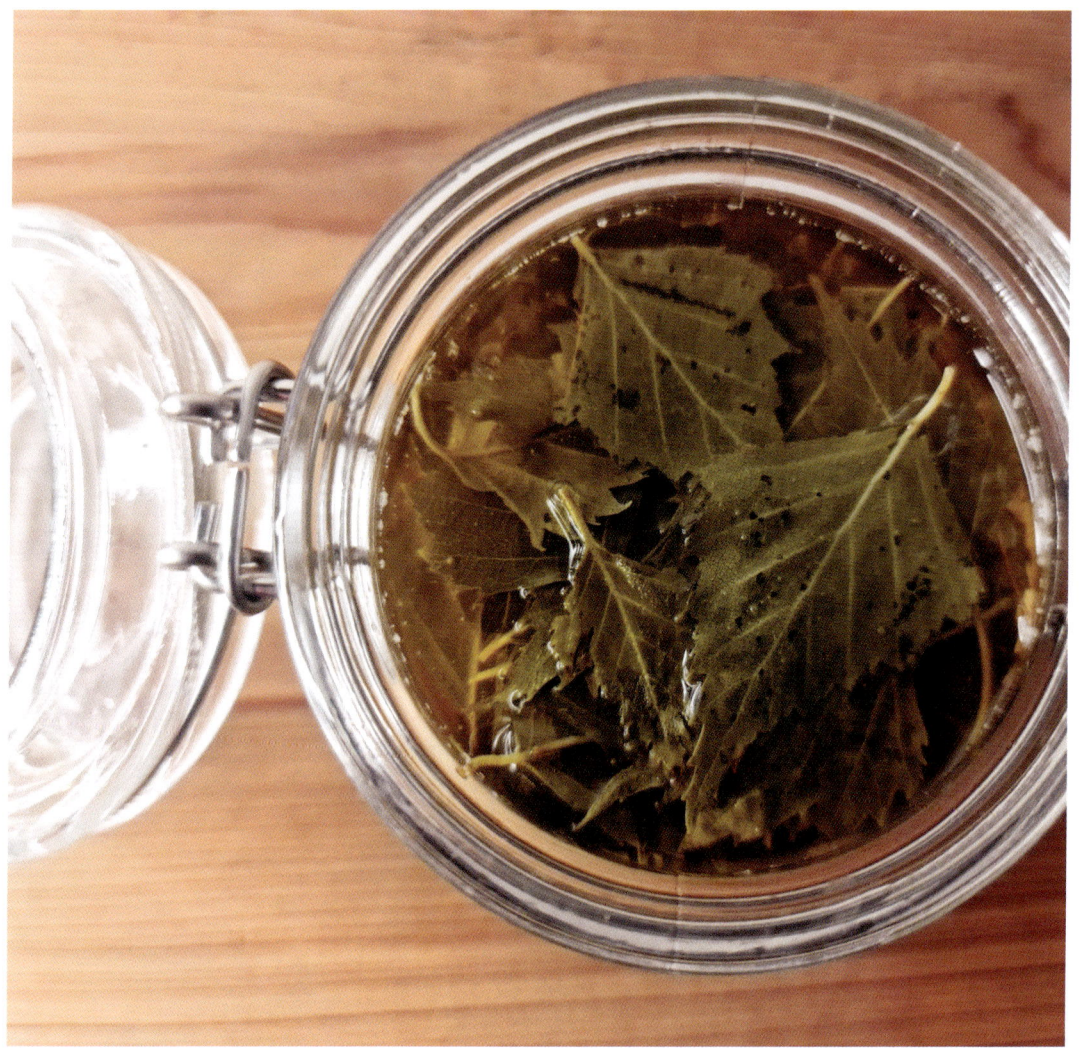

Pickled birch leaf

20g birch leaves
100ml cider vinegar
15g sugar
5g salt

Put the birch leaves and vinegar in pan and heat gently for about 10 minutes. Then add the sugar and salt. Let the sugar and salt dissolve, then allow the mixture to cool and place into a sterilised jar. Don't put the lid on until it has fully cooled down.

Pickled brambles

100g brambles
80ml cider vinegar
10g sugar
5g salt

Put the brambles and vinegar into a pan and heat gently until the brambles break down. Then add the sugar and salt. Let the sugar and salt dissolve, then allow the mixture to cool and place into a sterilised jar. Don't put the lid on until it has fully cooled down.

Pickled rowan berries

100g rowan berries
80ml cider vinegar
15g sugar
5g salt

Please use rowan berries that have been either frozen or, if fresh, boiled for 15 minutes.

Put the rowan berries and vinegar in a pan and heat gently until the rowan berries break down. Then add the sugar and salt. Let the sugar and salt dissolve, then allow the mixture to cool and place into a sterilised jar. Don't put the lid on until it has fully cooled down.

Foraged Condiments

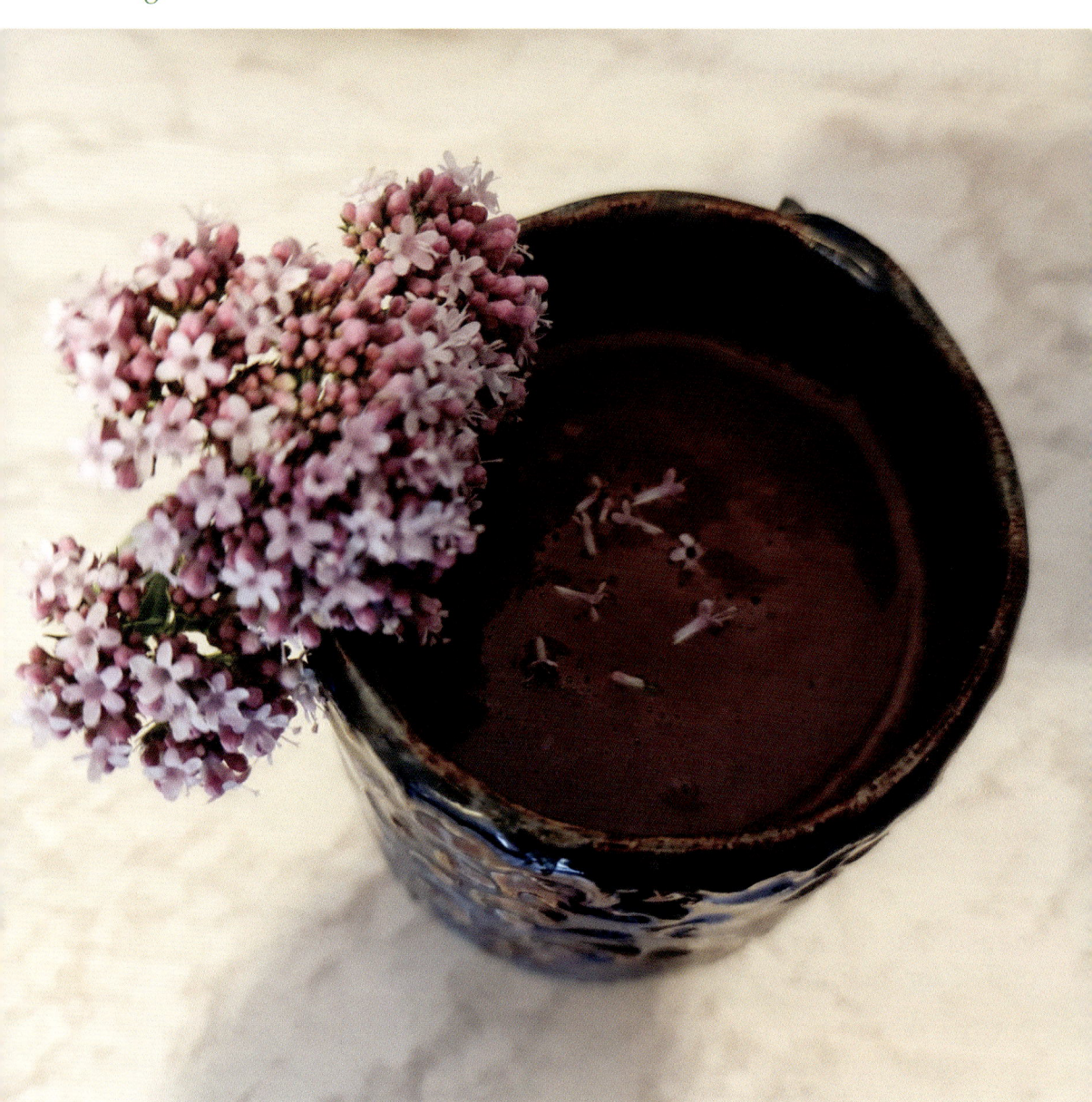

Hot drinks and a rob

Valerian hot chocolate

200ml milk of your choice (cow, goat or plant)
25g good-quality dark chocolate
10g sweetener (coconut sugar, honey, date syrup or maple syrup)
1g valerian root

Put the milk and chocolate (in small pieces or shavings) in a pan and heat until the chocolate is melted. Add the valerian and sugar or your choice, and very gently heat until the sugar is melted. Remove from the heat, strain out the valerian root and serve.

Foraged Condiments

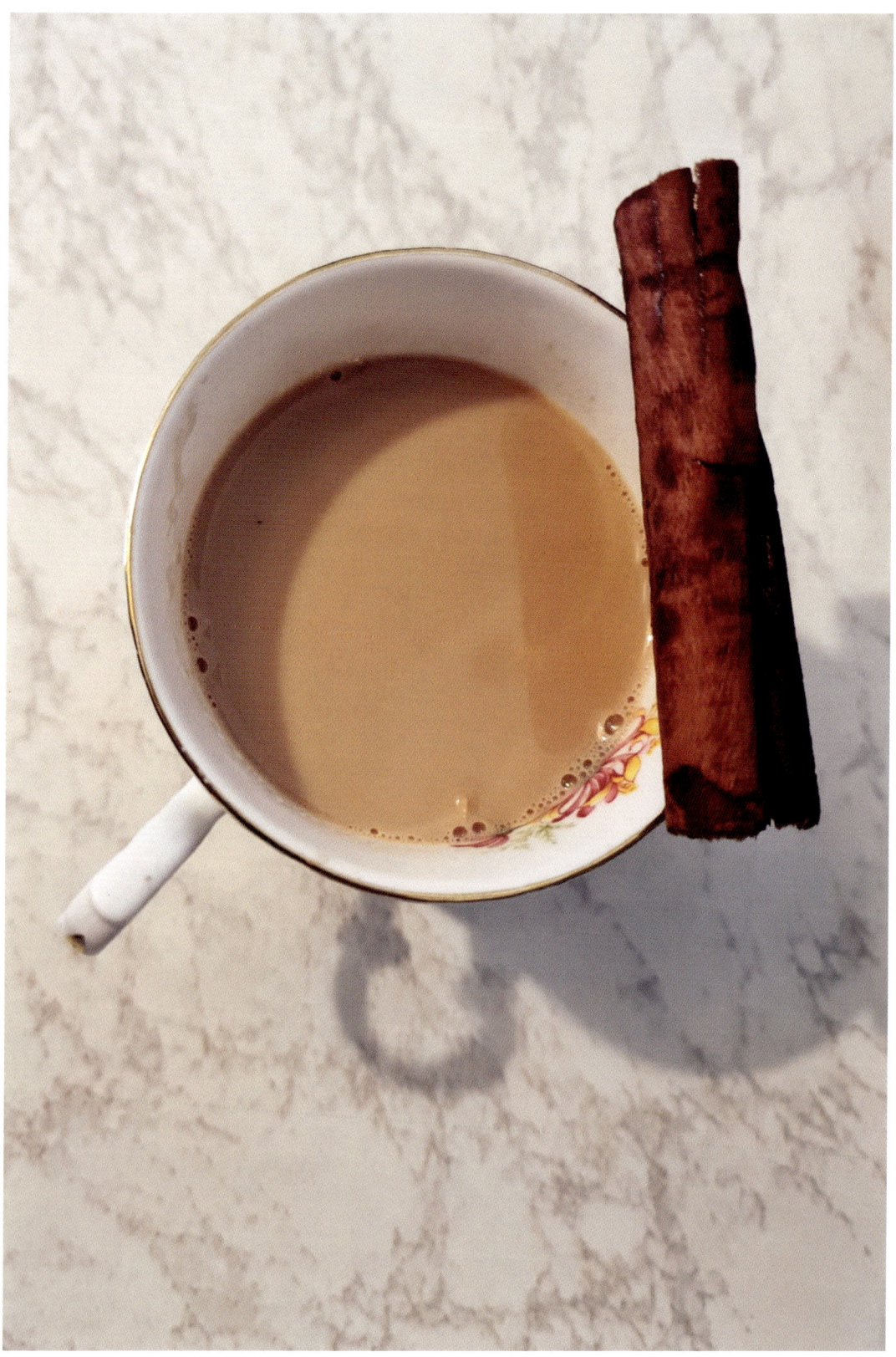

Chaga chai

200ml milk of your choice
10g chaga
1 black tea bag
2 cardamom seed pods
Half a teaspoon cinnamon
2g fresh ginger (or half a teaspoon of dried)
Pinch of black pepper
A tiny pinch of sea salt

Put the milk of your choice and all the other ingredients into a small pan. Gently heat to a rolling boil, then immediately take it down to a simmer and remove the tea bag.

Some people prefer to allow the chai to sit for a while until cool, then strain all herbs and spices as this gives a stronger, more robust flavour. Or, if preferred, you can just strain the hot mixture and drink.

Foraged Condiments

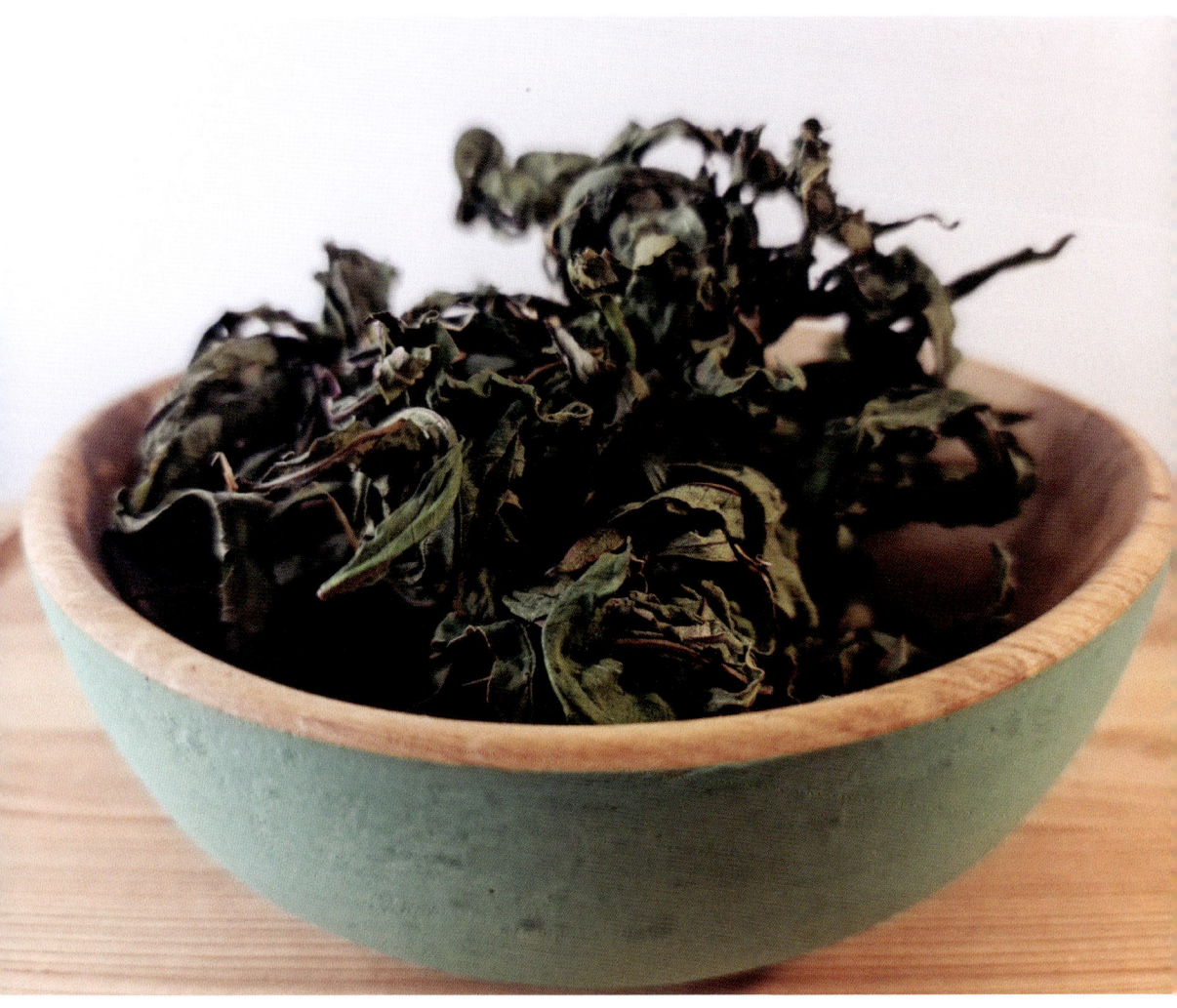

Ivan chai

Plenty of Rosebay willow leaves, allowed to dry and wilt overnight (I tend to use about 10 plants' worth at a time – I don't drink a lot of tea, though).

Scrunch up small handfuls of the leaves together into loose balls. Place these in an area where they won't be disturbed and loosely cover, but allowing airflow. For the next few days check them and move then around so no mould grows on them. They will start to lose the grassy smell and begin to turn black. Then they need to finished off in an oven or dehydrator. Use a low heat in both and go slowly.

Foraged Condiments

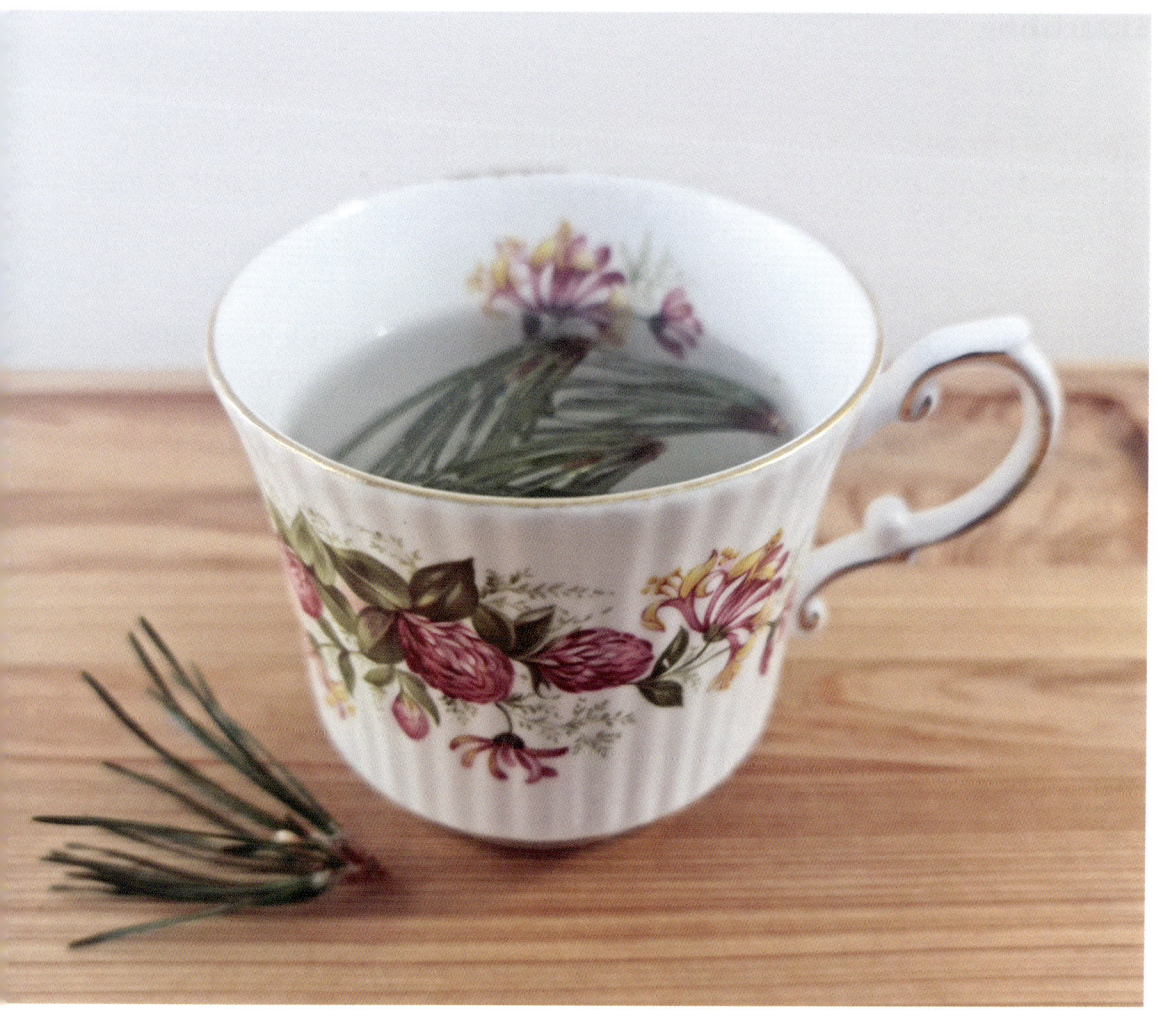

Pine needle tea

3 sprigs of pine needles
Hot water

Place the pine needles into a cup. Pour on near-boiling water and allow to steep for 10 minutes.

Elderberry rob

100g elderberries (off the stalk with no stalks included)
80g sugar
Half a cinnamon stick
1 star anise
3 cloves

Put the elderberries in a pan and cover with water. Bring to the boil and cook for 10 minutes. Then add the sugar and spices. Allow to cook for another 10 minutes or until it starts become syrupy. Strain well and place in a sterilised bottle. Keep in the fridge.

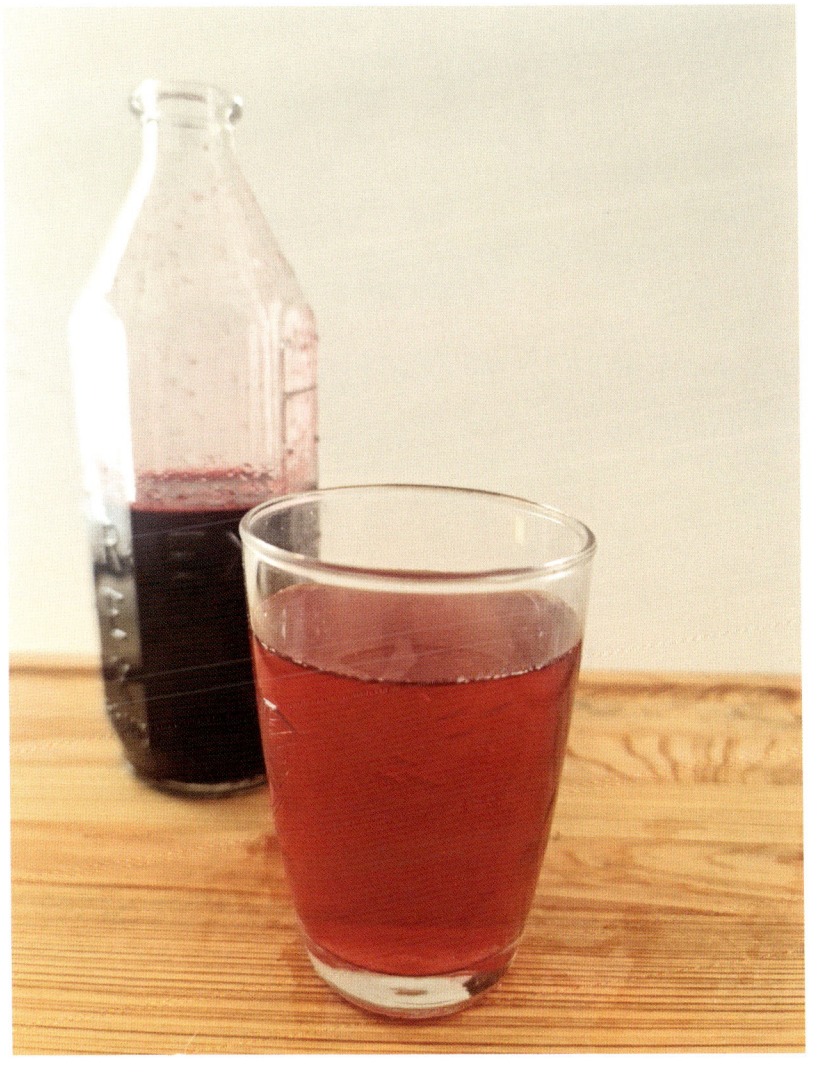

Foraged Condiments

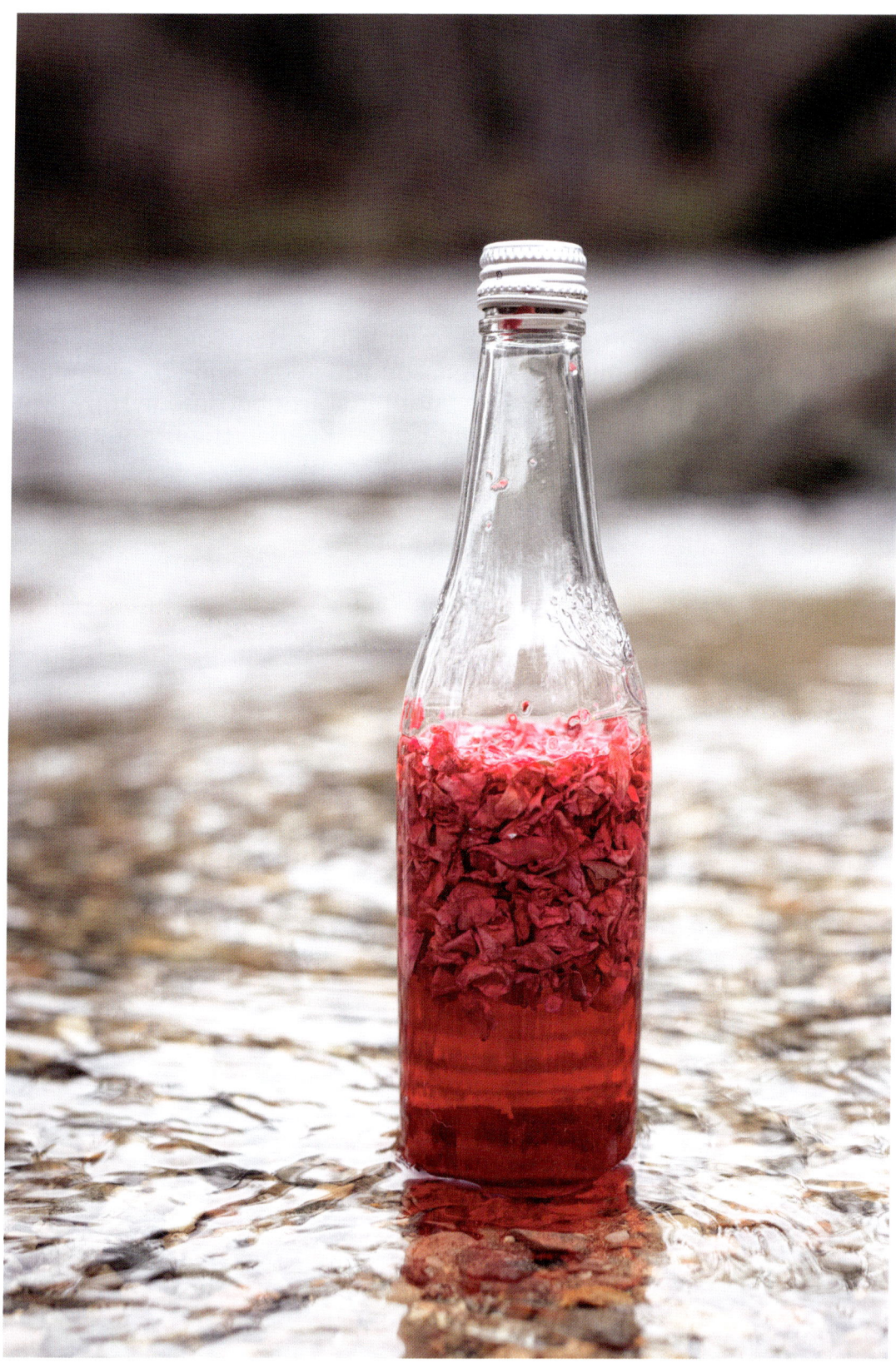

Tonic waters

Antigin tonic

5g chamomile flowers
5g lime flowers
2g rose petals

Remove about a third of the contents of a full 500ml tonic water bottle and set aside. Add the chamomile, lime flowers and rose petals. A funnel can help. Top up any gaps with the set-aside tonic, making sure all plant material is covered, and put the lid back on. Let it sit for two to three days. Strain the tonic, into a sterilised bottle and keep in the fridge. Note that when you open it will be very fizzy.

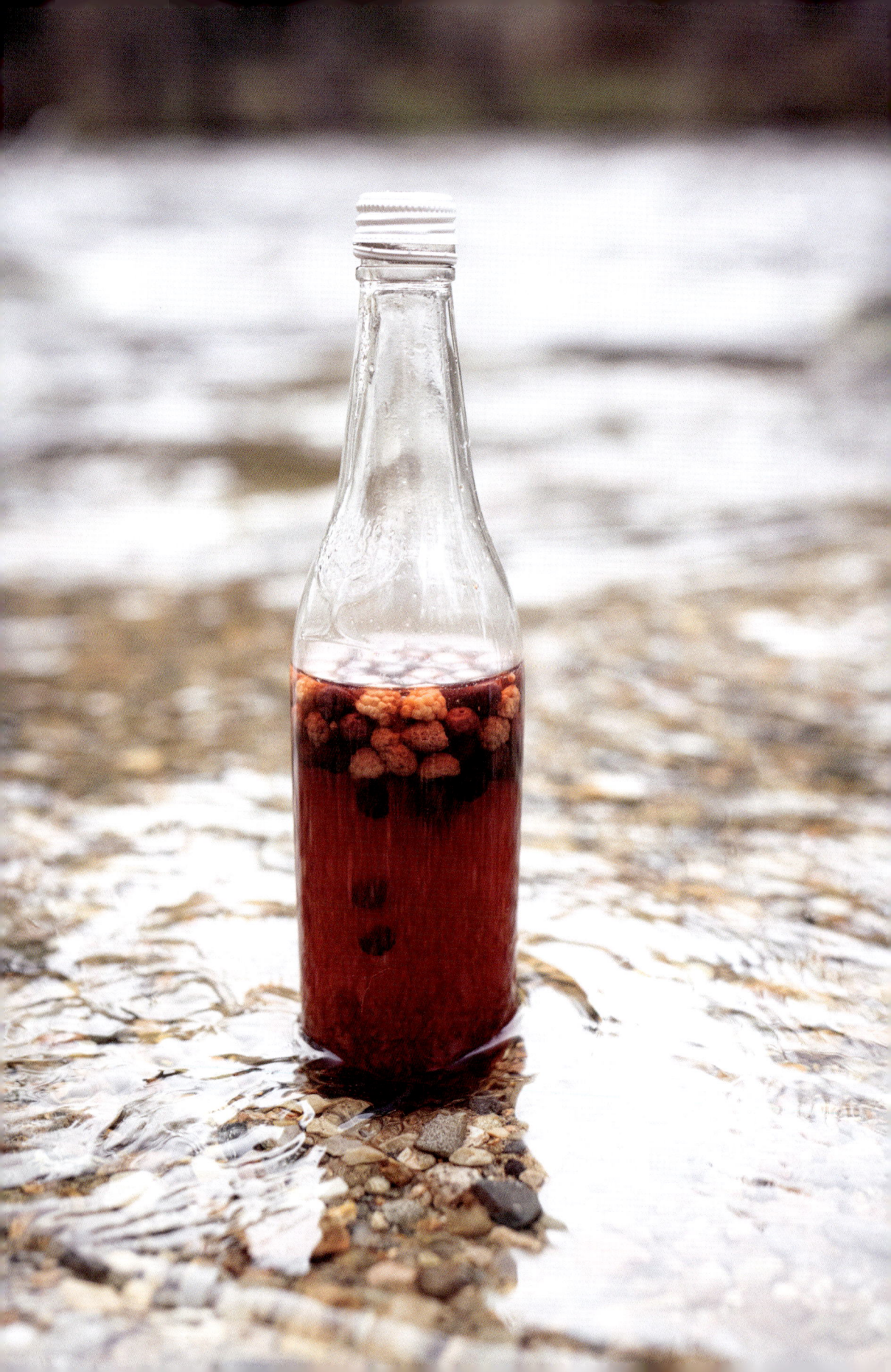

Berry tonic

5g raspberries
5g blaeberries/blueberries

Remove about a third of the contents of a full 500ml tonic water bottle and set aside. Add the raspberries and blaeberries. A funnel can help get them into the bottle. Then top up with the set-aside tonic, making sure all the berries are covered, and put the lid back on. Let it sit for two to three days. Strain the tonic into a sterilised bottle and keep in the fridge. Note that when you open it, it will be very fizzy.

Rose tonic

10g rose petals

Remove about a third of the contents of a full 500ml tonic water bottle and set aside. Add the rose petals. A funnel can help get them into the bottle. Then top up with the set-aside tonic, making sure all the berries are covered, and put the lid back on. Let it sit for two to three days. Strain the tonic into a sterilised bottle and keep in the fridge. Note that when you open it, it will be very fizzy.

Foraged Condiments

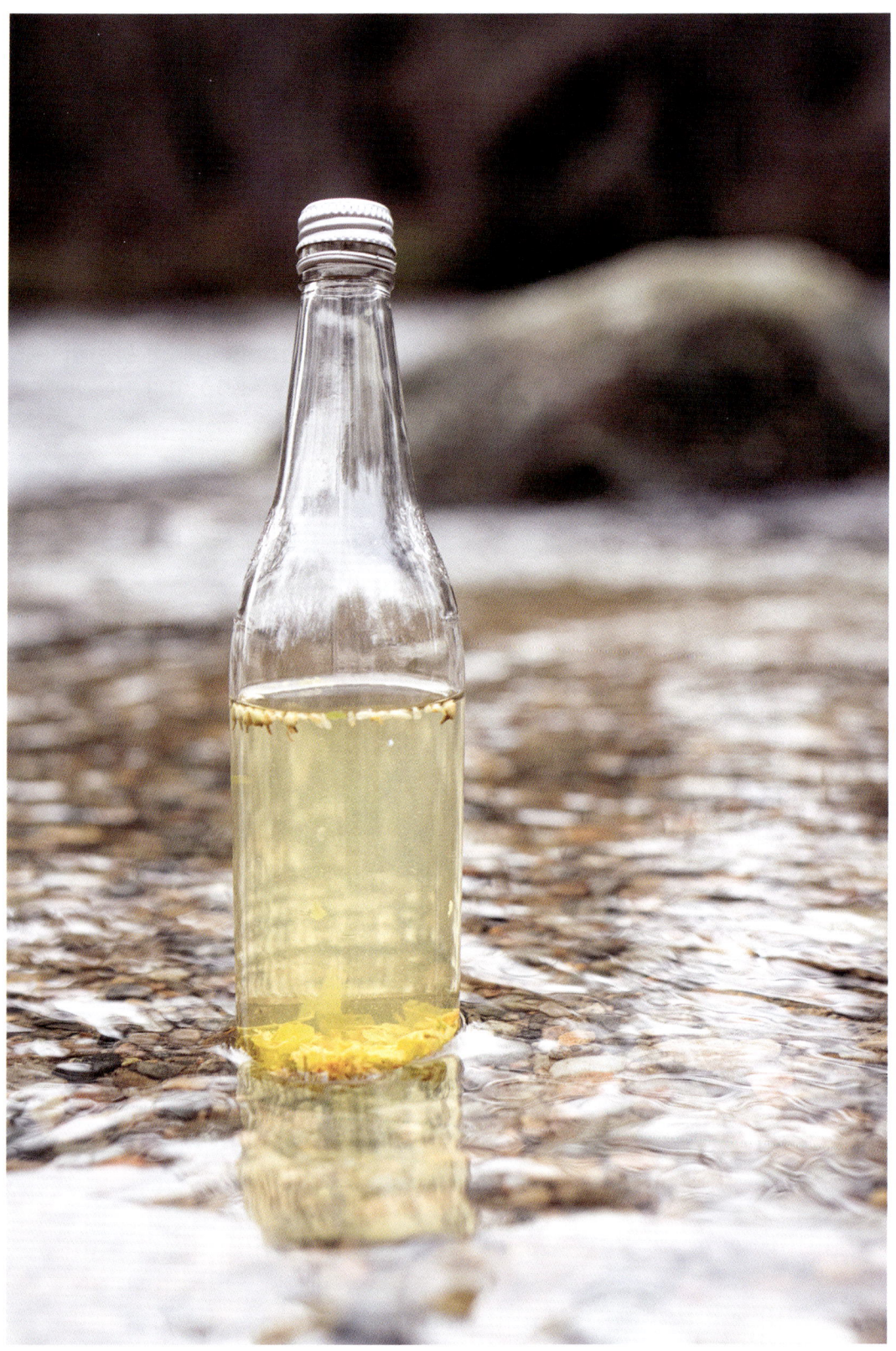

Lime flower tonic

10g lime flowers

Remove about a third of the contents of a full 500ml tonic water bottle and set aside. Add the lime flowers. A funnel can help get them into the bottle. Then top up with the set-aside tonic, making sure all the berries are covered, and put the lid back on. Let it sit for two to three days. Strain the tonic into a sterilised bottle and keep in the fridge. Note that when you open it, it will be very fizzy.

Foraged Condiments

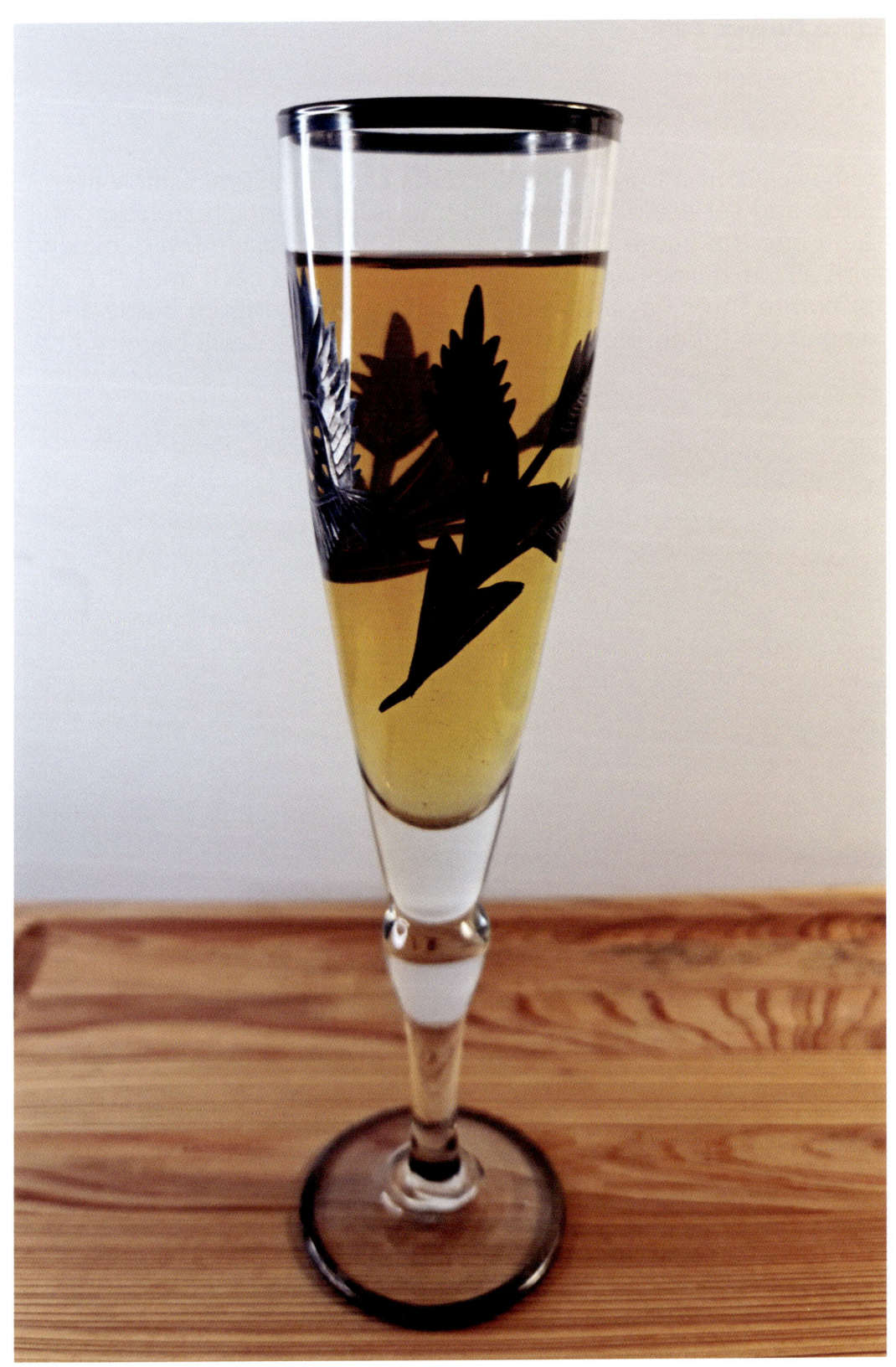

Vermouths

Foraged vermouth

10g chamomile or pineapple mayweed
5g meadowsweet
10g lime flower
3g yarrow
Bottle white wine, 750ml
250ml rosehip syrup

Open the bottle of white wine and remove about a third of the bottle, setting this aside for later. Put the rest in a small pan and add the herbs. bring the wine and herbs to a simmer very, very gently and slowly, then immediately remove from the heat. leave ove night to infuse. In the morning strain the herbs from the wine, place the wine and rosehip syrup together and mix well. Pour the infused wine and syrup into the original bottle or a newly sterilised bottle, then top up with the set-aside wing. Put the lid back on and shake to mix well.

Foraged Condiments

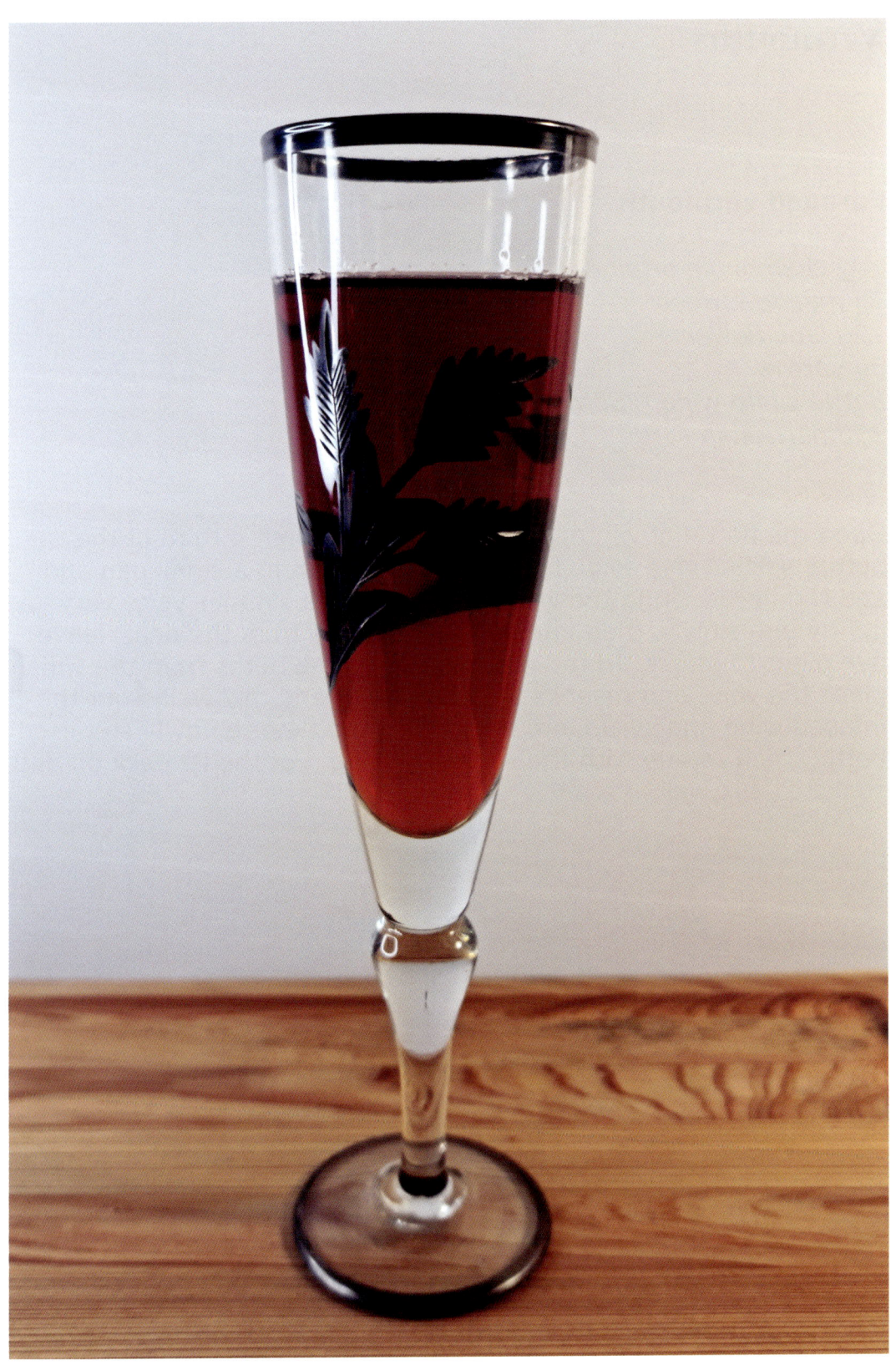

Antiviral vermouth

10g chamomile
3g yarrow
10g orange peel
Half a stick cinnamon
2 star anise
Bottle red wine, 750ml
250ml rose hip syrup

Open the bottle of red wine and remove about a third of the bottle, setting this aside for later. Put the rest in a small pan and add the herbs. Bring the wine and herbs to a simmer very, very gently and slowly, then immediately remove from the heat. Leave overnight to infuse. In the morning strain the herbs from the wine, place the wine and rosehip syrup together and mix well. Pour the infused wine and syrup into the original bottle or a newly sterilised bottle, then top up with the set-aside wine. Put the lid back on and shake to mix well.

Foraged Condiments

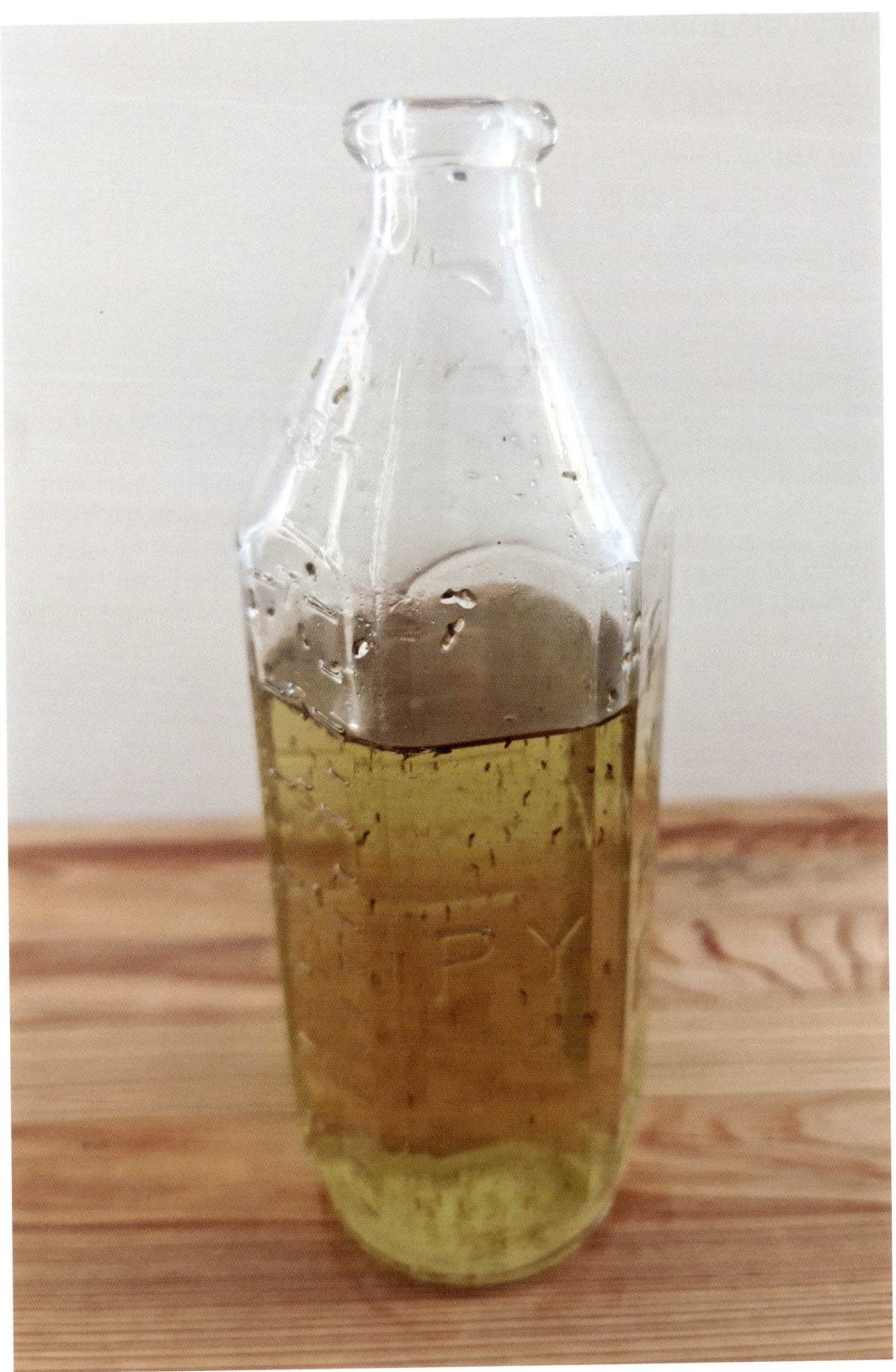

Syrups

Pineapple mayweed syrup

50g pineapple mayweed flowers, including stalks
150g sugar
Peel 1 lemon or 5g citric acid
300ml water

Put the pineapple mayweed flowers and water in a small pan. Bring to rolling boil then back to a simmer. Then add the sugar, allow it to dissolve gently. Remove from the heat, allow to cool and then strain. Add the lemon juice or citric acid. Pour into a sterilised jar or bottle and keep in the fridge.

Hogweed seed syrup

25g hogweed seeds
150g sugar
Peel 1 lemon or 5g citric acid
300ml water

Put the hogweed seeds and water in a small pan. Bring to rolling boil then back to a simmer. Then add the sugar, allow it to dissolve gently. Remove from the heat, allow to cool and then strain. Add the lemon juice or citric acid. Pour into a sterilised jar or bottle and keep in the fridge.

Foraged Condiments

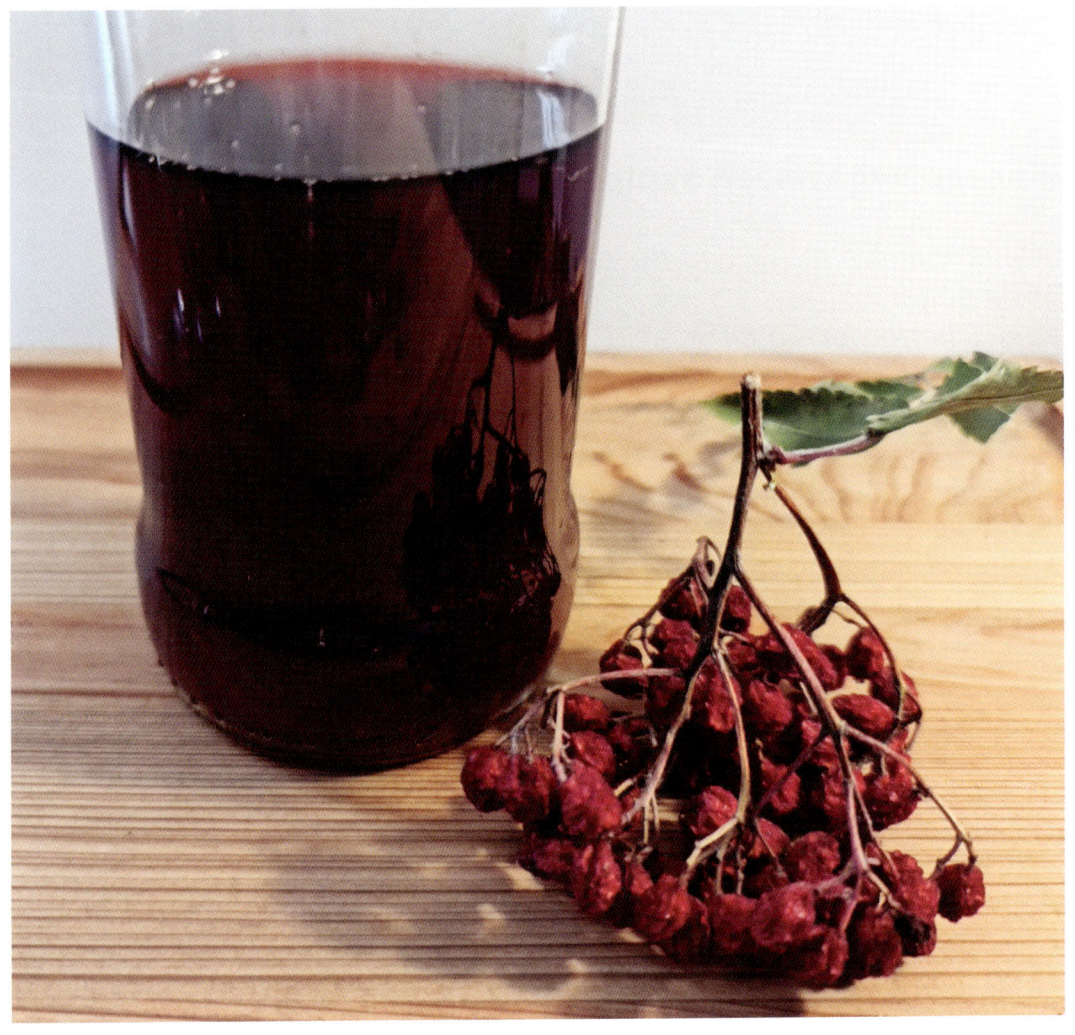

Rowan berry syrup

250g rowan berries
150g sugar
Peel 1 lemon or 5g citric acid
300ml water

Put the rowan berries and water in a small pan. Bring to rolling boil for 10 minutes then back to a simmer. Then add the sugar, allow it to dissolve gently. Remove from the heat, allow to cool and then strain. Add the lemon juice or citric acid. Pour into a sterilised jar or bottle and keep in the fridge.

Rosehip syrup

250g fresh rosehips, with all seeds and hairs removed
150g sugar
Peel 1 lemon or 5g citric acid
300ml water

Put the rosehips and water in a small pan. Bring to rolling boil then back to a simmer. Then add the sugar, allow it to dissolve gently. Remove from the heat, allow to cool and then strain. Add the lemon juice or citric acid. Pour into a sterilised jar or bottle and keep in the fridge.

Bramble syrup

250g brambles
150g sugar
Peel 1 lemon or 5g citric acid
300ml water

Put the brambles and water in a small pan. Bring to rolling boil then back to a simmer. Then add the sugar, allow it to dissolve gently. Remove from the heat, allow to cool and then strain. Add the lemon juice or citric acid. Pour into a sterilised jar or bottle and keep in the fridge.

Foraged Condiments

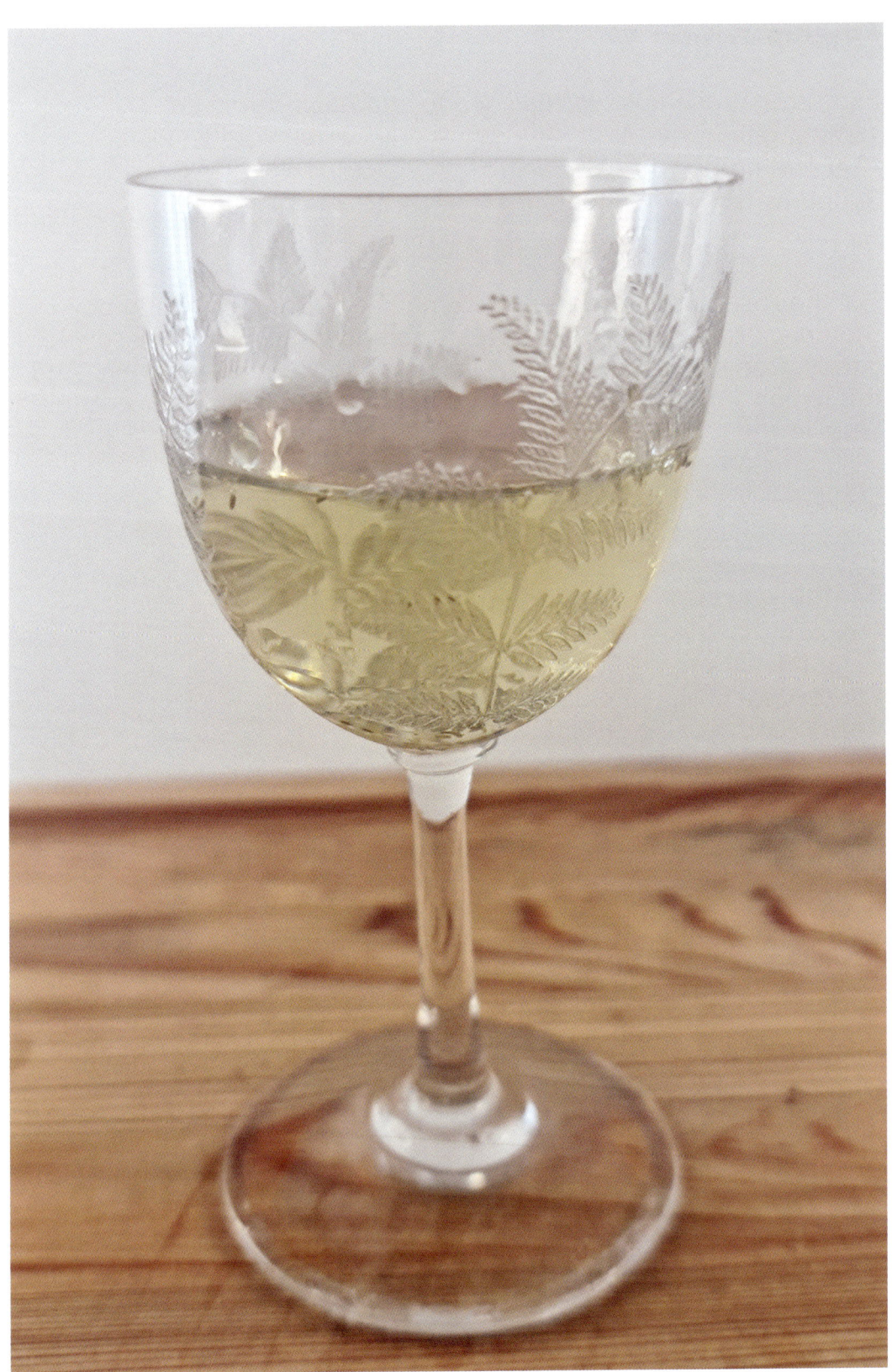

Pineapple mayweed infused vodka

Simply take a bottle of vodka and add sprigs of pineapple mayweed. Let it infuse for a week or two. Then strain.

Foraged Condiments

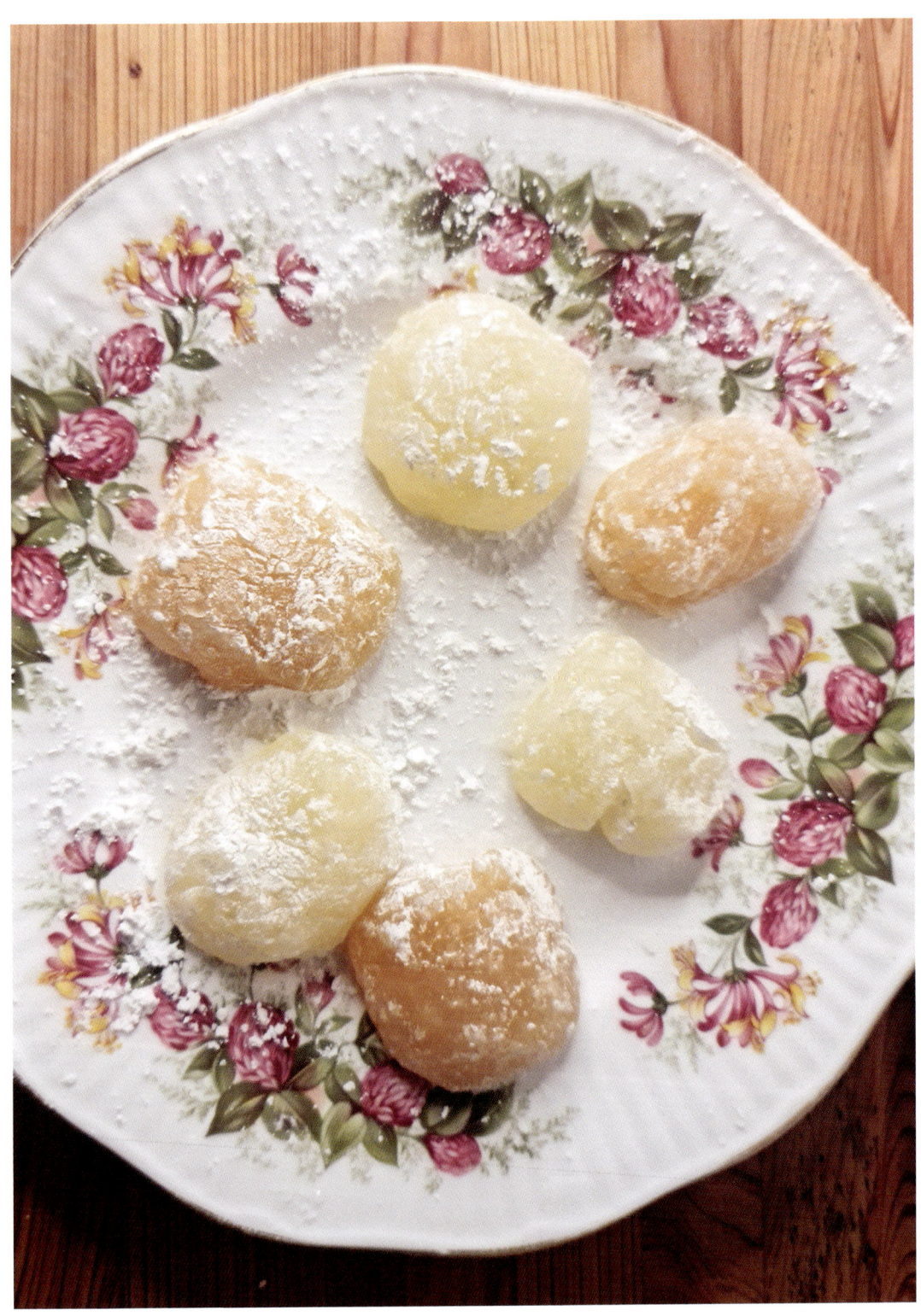

Turkish delights

Hawthorn Turkish delight

500g sugar
500ml water
Half a teaspoon cream of tartar
120g cornflour
2 tablespoons hawthorn syrup
Icing sugar and cornflour for dusting

Have a shallow oiled dish ready.

Put the sugar and water in a pan and add the cream of tartar. Boil for 10 to 15mins until it starts to go syrupy. Ideally it should reach 115°C to 118°C.

In a separate bowl add cold water to the cornflour and mix thoroughly. Then add into the sugar syrup, whisking all the time. It will eventually start to come away at the sides of the pan. You should be able to see a line drawn in it with a spatula.

This should take about 20 minutes, but don't leave it though. Stay and watch it. Also be careful as this mixture can create bubbles that are hot when they burst. Stir in the syrup well and then transfer to the oiled dish. Allow to flatten and cool.

It will be ready in about 24 hours. Dust icing sugar and cornflour on the pieces you cut.

Pineapple mayweed Turkish delight

500g sugar
500ml water
Half a teaspoon cream of tartar
120g cornflour
2 tablespoons pineapple mayweed syrup
Icing sugar and cornflour for dusting

Have a shallow oiled dish ready.

Put the sugar and water in a pan and add the cream of tartar. Boil for 10 to 15mins until it starts to go syrupy. Ideally it should reach 115°C to 118°C.

In a separate bowl add cold water to the cornflour and mix thoroughly. Then add into the sugar syrup, whisking all the time. It will eventually start to come away at the sides of the pan. You should be able to see a line drawn in it with a spatula.

This should take about 20 minutes, but don't leave it though. Stay and watch it. Also be careful as this mixture can create bubbles that are hot when they burst. Stir in the syrup well and then transfer to the oiled dish. Allow to flatten and cool.

It will be ready in about 24 hours. Dust icing sugar and cornflour on the pieces you cut.

Foraged Condiments

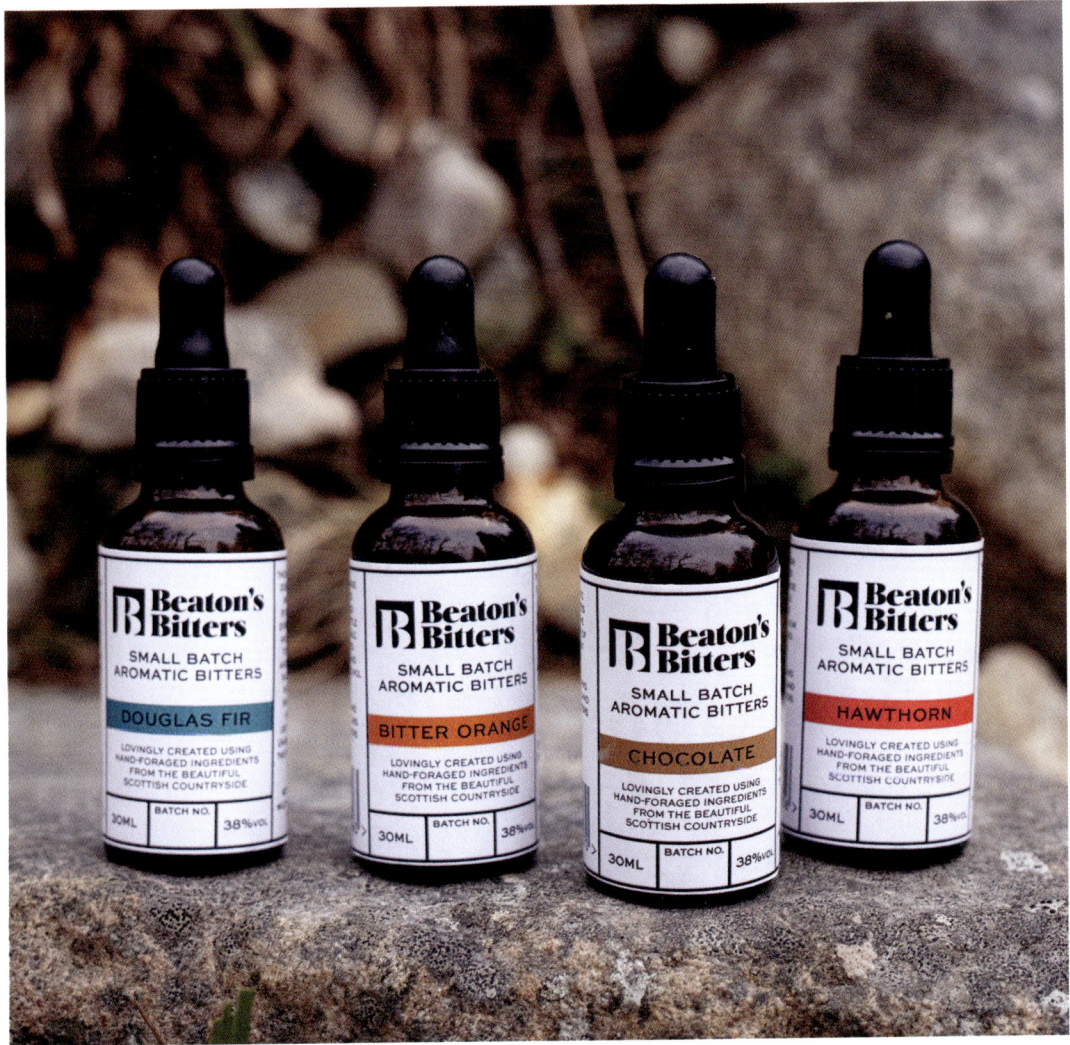

Bitters

Orange bitters

100ml vodka
5g orange peel
3g yarrow
5g chamomile
3g dandelion leaf
1 star anise
3 cloves

Put the vodka and herbs and spices into a sterilised jar. Place the lid on it and allow to sit for two weeks. Strain and pour into sterilised dropper bottles.

Chocolate bitters

100ml vodka
10g chocolate nibs
3g yarrow
1g bogbean
5g lime flowers

Put the vodka and herbs and spices into a sterilised jar. Place the lid on it and allow to sit for two weeks. Strain and pour into sterilised dropper bottles.

Douglas fir bitters

100ml vodka
10g Douglas fir needles
3g yarrow
5g lime flowers
5g grapefruit peel

Put the vodka and herbs and spices into a sterilised jar. Place the lid on it and allow to sit for two weeks. Strain and pour into sterilised dropper bottles.

Hawthorn bitters

100ml vodka
10g hawthorn berry pulp
5g chamomile
5g hibiscus
3g lime flowers
3g dandelion leaf

Put the vodka and herbs and spices into a sterilised jar. Place the lid on it and allow to sit for two weeks. Strain and pour into sterilised dropper bottles.

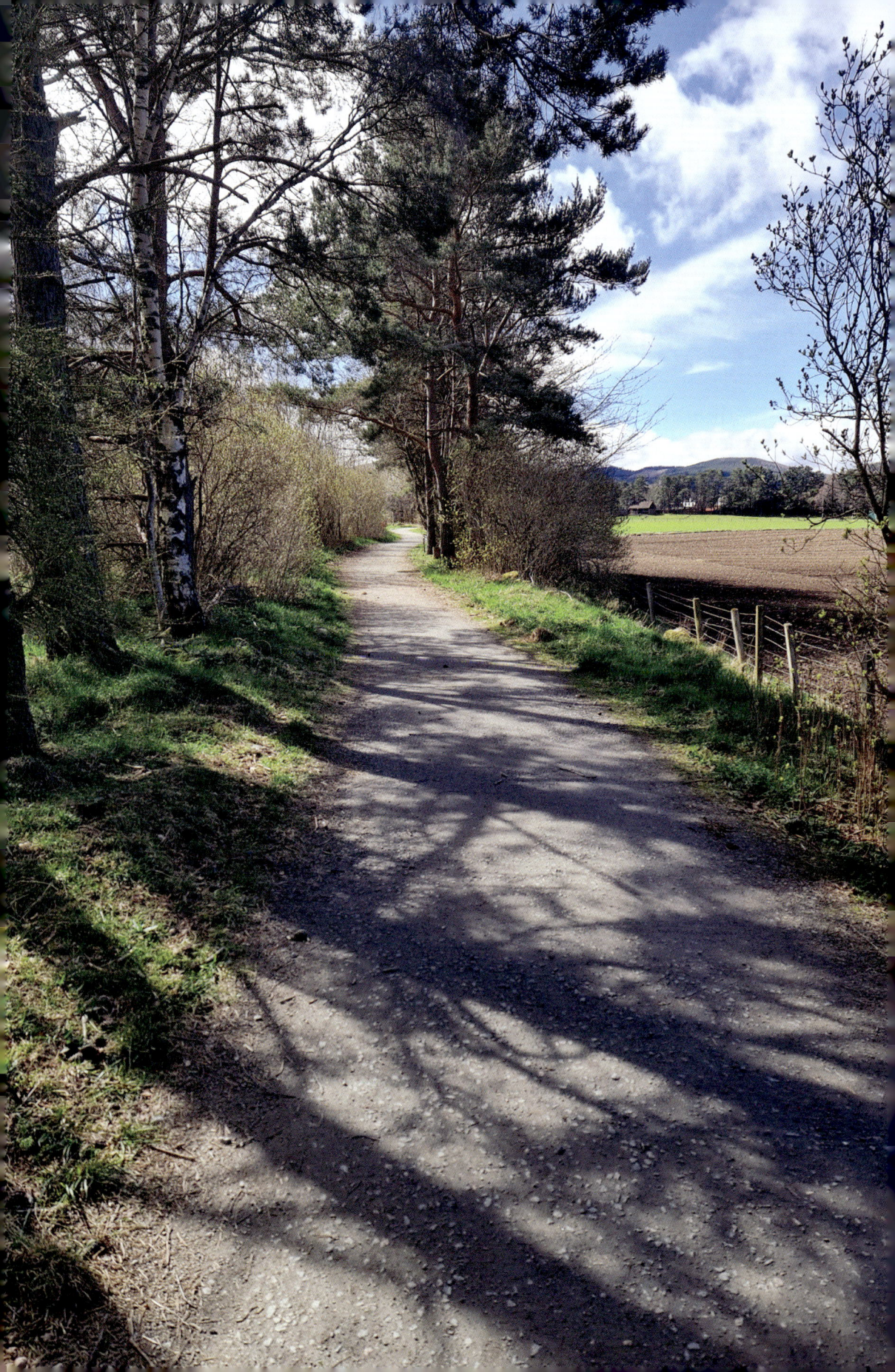

alone watching the start of the plants coming back after Winter and the joy that brings.

As I start to feel the deadline looming of only eating wild food I can feel an anxiety around where am I going to get my food from. Obviously by going to go out and getting foraged wild greens. I'm in the Cairngorms in Scotland and our cohort for the study starts at the beginning of April. Will there be enough wild greens coming through?

This experiment is with 25 other people in various locations throughout the UK. We have a few online meetings to discuss how to do the study, including how to use the Zoe equipment required, namely the blood sugar monitor, the stool sample and finger prick test. We have an app for messages between us as a group, and we have a dedicated room on another app for online meetings, the Zoe app and the blood sugar monitor app. Communications are good. We had a meeting last night between a few of us to discuss what our thoughts were about each meal of the day. It was interesting as we all had different variations in the way we eat. I like a hearty breakfast but don't eat that much during the day until early evening, when I have a full dinner or snack sometimes in the evening when most of my work is done. Others skip breakfast and wait until later in the day to eat. Others are doing intermittent fasting.

We all of course have various dietary requirements and preferences. I'm lactose intolerant, so giving up dairy for this study is not an issue for me. Others have dairy as a main part of their daily diet. For me giving up my usual vegetables will be difficult. I predict I will miss leafy green vegetables the most, but thankfully for me that is simply a changeover to the wild greens.

I love potatoes and eat them frequently through the week. Oats I eat an inordinate amount of – porridge for breakfast with various topping and additions, and oatcakes for snacks. One of the thoughts in the informal meeting was: are we just replacing things we eat now with a wild form? For example, oatcakes for acorn pancakes or chestnut pancakes. This has thrown up loads of questions and interesting aspects far more than just swapping out your diet and where it comes from.

What if all our supply lines stopped, say if we were in a war zone, or what happens when quite regularly a crop fails? Yes, we live without that crop for that season. We have had plenty of times when crops have failed and prices go up.

It has really got me thinking. We don't think of our food supply coming from around

Foraged Condiments

us, as there is so much travel involved in our food. So to be searching out our food really locally by eating the wild plants around us is interesting and scary at the same time.

I know where the local patches of nettle are, but will they be enough to sustain me? Here is where part of the thinking changes. A small amount from the nettle patch, a small amount of dandelion leaves, woodrush, jack in the hedge, plantain, ground elder and wild garlic will give me a meal without depleting the patches of each plant. The bulk of my wild food is going to come from venison and fish.

As mentioned, we are all being tested beforehand for our gut microbiome, blood fat and sugar levels. This involves taking samples of stool and blood two weeks before the start and wearing a blood glucose monitor for two weeks. At the beginning of this we did a day's test involving eating specially made muffins from Zoe and fasting for four hours, then another set of muffins, fasting for two hours.

Now I feel I have really started this project. I can feel a panic rising, so I start to think about what food I need to gather and prepare. My food hoarding tendencies set in. I start to seek out the foods I can store in the freezer, venison and fish. I have a stock of wild plants dried and some wild condiments, some of which are suitable as they only contain wild ingredients.

I nervously went and looked at the local patches of plants local to me. They are starting to come up, but what stage will they be in April? That will depend on a few factors like daylight hours, warmth, rain and sunshine.

I suddenly feel like I'm an ancient hunter and gatherer, where the seasons and weather matter a whole lot more than just what am I wearing for today's weather. Now it's when will I get to eat nettles without destroying the growth of that particular patch so that I have some later in the year. Also we live in a community – I don't own that patch, so anyone can come along and take plants from it.

Now I feel vulnerable and ill at ease with my food supply. I do have dried nettles in the cupboard, so I feel safer. I'm not a competition person, and working in a team and collaboratively is much more my ways. Most people locally don't see nettles and all the other spring greens as food.
The notable exception is wild garlic, and a few years ago I saw a significant portion

of a wild garlic patch hacked to the ground. No thought was given for the plant surviving and producing flowers and seeds for reproduction. My heart sank that day. There is a lot for modern humans to learn about how to look after the planet and to not think of just themselves.

It did prompt me to teach more earnestly about how to respect the plants and their growth areas and ability to reproduce for next year and coming years. But this is now worrying me for my own supply, but that makes me selfish.

Time to stop worrying, and get on and prepare.

Preparation involves working out the parameters of the study and what can be obtained for it. I have some plants dried and some apples and berries dried from last year. We are allowed to buy food in that is wild. So I start searching and looking for ingredients. I found a few places, frantically order and hope it arrives in time.

The whole change of supply makes me feel nervous. There were a few places to buy wild produce online, and I got all excited about one place as I found a product that was venison and wild boar … I got disappointed when I realised it was a can of dog food. It is easier to buy wild food for dogs than it is for humans.

The search needed to be widened. Living where I do there are plenty of deer on the hills, and we found someone to help us. If I was doing this for longer then I would have learnt how to stalk and shoot a deer. Maybe I will do that in the future.

Fishing is something I have some experience of and enjoy. I learnt to fish on Lewis where neighbours showed me the basics. Off I went into the interior of the island to find brown trout in the freshwater lochs. It was a good walk out and back. A few brownies for dinner were usually found from each time. There's nothing better than fresh trout.

In those days it felt like I had more time in a day than I do now. So venison and now some wild boar secured by Katy – I'm starting to feel more relaxed. Fish will come from the fish van, and if it was open the new fishmongers opening in Ballater soon. That will be at the end of April, so just as I'm finishing.

Then as ingredients start to arrive and merge with what stocks I already have I start to prep and bring all the ingredients together in my cupboards. This involves also going to local plant patches I know with Katy so we can see what stage the plants are at. It feels different from most Springs as we are going to be relying on these patches for our dinner.

There is still a feeling of delight seeing the plants growing and thriving. Attending collective video calls with folk in the project to hear how they have all been getting on has helped settle me. I'm getting ideas and hearing how folk are feeling. Now I'm starting to feel ready … why does the date feel like it is looming closer? Why has the excitement got a tinge of dread about it?

It's losing supply and comfort of that I think is giving me dread. We are more at the mercy of the elements. All our crops are always at mercy to the elements, but somehow we feel a sense of distance from that when we buy our food in supermarkets and online shops.

This new supply line has hardly any sense of distance, and that starts to make me feel better. I'm closer to our food and the seasons. I've always had a sense of the seasons. We all do, but working more closely the last decade or so has really helped me connect on a deeper level.

One of the greatest aspects of this project that wasn't put on paper is the great sense of community and caring for each other. It's an automatic caring nature for each other. We start tomorrow.

Day 1
I wake up feeling woefully unprepared then remember I have some cod that has thawed. Then I get a phone call while still in my bed thinking and planning for the day and the food I'll gather, prepare and eat. It's not an unusual aspect of the day for me, I love food and cooking.

The phone call is from Katy. She's outside with some venison and wild boar for the freezer. I'm there in a few minutes, so happy and grateful to Katy for finding, ordering and then delivering. How kind and at the moment very thoughtful as I haven't been out of the village for a while.

As I'm gently pushing the anxiety I've learned to do that in stages and keep some level of comfort for my nervousness until next time. All that aside, I'm ready to go out and find the plants I was thinking of to go with the cod. A great sign and for me and Yarrow the dog. We go with no hesitation from either of us.

My mood is a tad low and feel a bit flat. I manage my tasks but notice they are a bit harder today. I put it down to the flurry of the last few weeks. Breakfast was an organic egg and some nettle seed. Nettle seeds for me go really well with eggs. They have a slightly seaweedy and a deep mineral flavour. So it's not that an unusual breakfast, the difference being I have more time to prepare and eat.

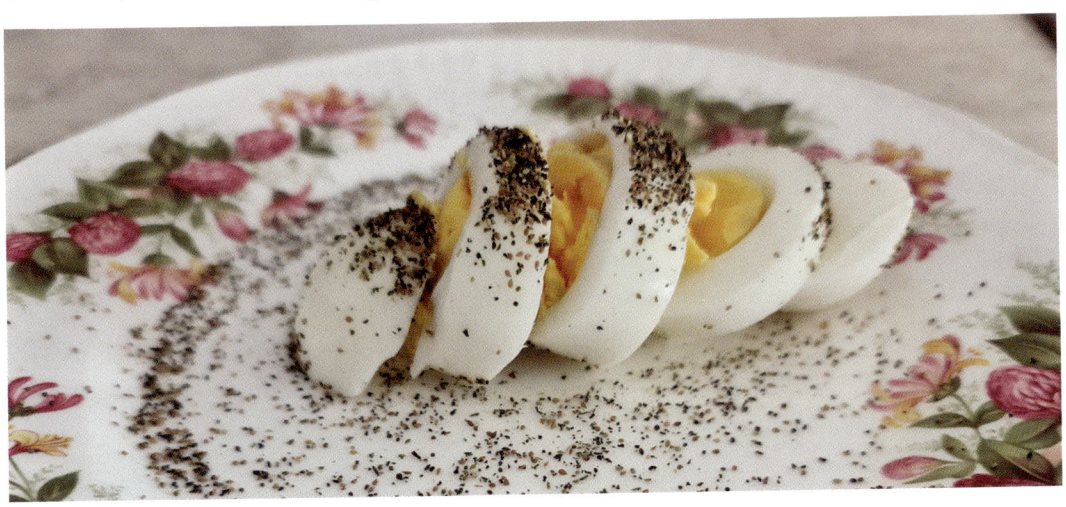

I often miss lunch and snack during the day as I'm working. If I'm out and about then I'll eat lunch, but being at home I snack until dinner time. That's what I do but the snacks have changed. They have become dried apple slices, hazelnuts, walnuts, dried blaeberries and dried wild raspberries. For dinner, the cod is wrapped in sweet cicely leaves, dipped in beaten egg and coated in chestnut flour. I cook it in the air fryer, and it is excellent. I really enjoy my first wild meal.

My evening snack is an organic apple. I relax with a satisfied feeling and fall asleep easily.

Day 2

I wake up tired but OK today. I have an activity planned with Katy – we're going birch sap tapping. I take my trusty antique hand-drill, a few plastic inserts and some bottles to help catch the sap. It will be collected tomorrow.

I'm slightly worried because it's a bit late in the year to be collecting birch sap, which is near the end of its season. So I'm not certain we will get anything. That's foraging – you don't always know you're going to get something. You work with the seasons and the conditions of that year. I like that. It makes you tune in a lot more to your own surroundings and environment.

This also shows that we're starting this experiment at the very beginning of spring. I have to say for this year it would have been better to have started a bit later. Saying that, there's a connection with how our ancestors must have felt after winter and trying to find enough food to eat. Will the stores that were collected later last year be enough to get us through to the abundance of late spring?

I've mostly lived in remote places and houses that were off the beaten track in one way or another, and preparing for times where it was hard to get food, whether that be a broken-down vehicle or snow or storm. I learned to have a store of food in. I actually really enjoyed this aspect of living remotely and I find it comforting to have a store of food in. But I don't have back-up food and stores for this project.

So essentially this is a year where ancestors' stores would not have made it through, and how do you survive then? Saying that. I haven't hunted the venison or the wild boar, and I haven't had time to go fishing. So we're starting with the early spring greens and, today, birch sap.

Day 3

I wake up tired. I'm having to run to the toilet and my bowels are loose. I now know why I felt low a couple of days ago. My period has started, and it's a heavy flow. I climb back into bed and pull the covers over my head. This is not the way I want to start this experiment. Of course, every month I have a period, but not as heavy or as energy-draining as this one.

But here we are and we'll have to get on with it. I decide to not go out for the day and to conserve some energy. I eat probably more of the usual snacks that I had yesterday. I can tell I'm using food as a comfort factor. My evening meal is the wild boar and fresh nettle stew from yesterday.

Katy informs me by WhatsApp there isn't enough birch sap. I suspected this would be the case. I got a flow of birch sap about two weeks ago, which I drank straight away, and didn't expect it to still be here as I've seen the beginning of the tips of the leaves growing.

For this experiment we have been allocated one jar of wild honey for the month.

Today we were hoping to get enough to make at least a bit of birch sap syrup, which is actually a lot of birch sap. You need one hundred litres to make one litre of birch sap syrup, but alas it isn't meant to be.

I like that we did the activity together, and it's Katy's first time so she gets to try it straight from the tree, just not how to make the syrup yet. I curl up into my bed and fall asleep easily.

Day 4

It's a day of desk work. I have patient prescriptions to create and send to the dispensary, letters to send to patients and the usual flurry of emails that so many of us have as a steady flow in our lives.

I feel really blessed to have a mental map of where good edible foraged food is close to my home. It is days like these where I'm focusing and folk are waiting that my mental map comes into its own. It has taken me years to build that map.

I am feeling a bit lazy today, so I opt for smoked mackerel and a simple salad. I go to a very local patch of dandelions and pick four young dandelion plants. This is with the root as well as the young fresh leaf greens. Opposite them is a good patch of young plantain. I pick a few of those leaves and hurry back home.

Digging up roots doesn't feel that good to me. I've actually chosen dandelions where I know there's an abundance of them in that place. It's on a public pathway, and I'm very careful how much I take. You don't want to diminish an area so that the plant dies out in that place.

When it comes to dandelion some people might want that to happen, but I don't. I want to be able to go back and enjoy some dandelion flowers later in the year. There are numerous insects that feed off the flowers early in the year – it's not just for my visual pleasure, it's for food for insects and bees.

To dig out roots on someone else's land you need their permission. Because once you dig up the root you have killed the whole plant. So I'm very aware of where I'm picking the dandelion roots, and I'm very aware of how many I'm taking at a time. I spread out my places and think quite hard about where I'm taking from.

I end up with a salad of dandelion leaves and plantain leaves with the delicious blaeberry vinegar. I roast the dandelion roots and add a touch of honey. When they're young like this they're delicious.

I like them in the autumn too. Roasted, they give a delicious caramelly chocolate coffee flavour without the caffeine. If I had time before starting this project I would have made pear and dandelion root chutney, which is delicious.

Day 5

It's apple slices for breakfast, and walnuts and hazelnuts for lunch. I'm getting on a roll and routine with this, and it feels good. It's another desk day as there's a lot of paperwork this week. I managed to get the majority of it done yesterday, so I have more time to go outside.

I go a bit further afield than I did yesterday. My mind can wander a bit more and think about where to find the plants I want to eat so that I'm not depleting patches close to the house. I want a new patch of dandelions essentially.

I go up the railway line and into the woods. Sure enough, I find young dandelions growing as I walk to a known nettle patch. I see some young yarrow leaves and a fresh patch of plantain. I start to think how many people in the village could live on this at this time of year. I'm also thinking about for later in the year and not take too much so there is enough for later – and that's without anyone else foraging this patch. Then that's just thinking of humans. Many insects and birds rely on these plants for their food. It's such an interconnected world, and we are only a part of it.

Day 6

It's boiled eggs and nettle seed for breakfast. I'm up early, which isn't like me as I'm a confirmed night owl, but today it's up and out to meet up with Katy. We are going to the seashore. The reason we're starting early is for the low tide, and we want to find seaweed.

The shore we're heading for is a good hour's drive. I was nervous before going to sleep about travelling, but I'm too sleepy in the morning to even have anxiety. It's a good sign. I get excited as we leave the village as I feel settled.

I love food. Normally on a day out I will be looking for places to get snacks and something a bit different to eat, but we can't do that today. This pains me slightly, but of course I've got a plethora of snacks with me. I have a couple of apples, some nuts and a boiled egg.

We arrive at the shoreline and get our bearings slightly. Neither of us have done this before. I have gone foraging for seaweed with other knowledgeable folk – but not on my own and not for my dinner. It feels a bit daunting but also exciting.

We muddle through with our collective knowledge, some of which was only learnt a few days ago. We find some kelp and move on to a different shoreline. There I find what I think is some pepper dulse. I am unsure of myself and even spend time looking at the shoreline plants to feel more confident and then go back. Yes, it is pepper dulse. I'm very pleased.

The dogs, Yarrow and Mac, are having a great time, running around and playing with seaweed themselves. Our lunch is the snacks that we brought, and Katie adds a hazelnut chestnut base for an apple tart that she had made the day before. It tastes so good as we share it together.

On our way home we went past a wild garlic patch. Of course we stopped. I showed Katy the difference between bluebell leaves, lords and ladies leaves and wild garlic leaves. You don't want to get those mixed up. So we continue to gather a few leaves for our dinner and the next few days. Wild garlic keeps well in the fridge.

I look up from my selecting leaves and I see someone had just cut through a whole plant. My heart sinks. I stop my initial reaction, which was one of noooo!, and gently explain that that plant won't grow back now and we don't harvest this way.

I show her how to take a few leaves respectfully for the continuity of life of the plant. If we take with just ourselves in mind for that temporary moment of one meal and we go back to that patch there won't be anything left for us, let alone the needs of the insects and other animals, and the interconnection of the plants.

We can't continue if we harvest without thought and respect. Our world is set up that thinking just of ourselves is almost encouraged and not questioned very much. We need to start seeing ourselves as part of nature, not separate from it.

I get home and have two smoked mackerel as a snack. And then I make a venison, rosehip and wild garlic stew. While that is cooking I deal with the seaweed we got today. I wash it and place it in the dehydrator. This in turn causes my house to smell of seaweed for a day or two while preserving the seaweed for a later date.

Day 7

After the usual eggs and nettle seed for breakfast it's another writing and paperwork day. So I'm at my desk most of the time, but I need to find a balance between achieving all my tasks and getting my food. Today I feel like I achieved a bit of that balance.

I end up going further afield to collect from different patches. I go deeper into the woods and find a really healthy patch of nettles. I take a few of the tops and bring

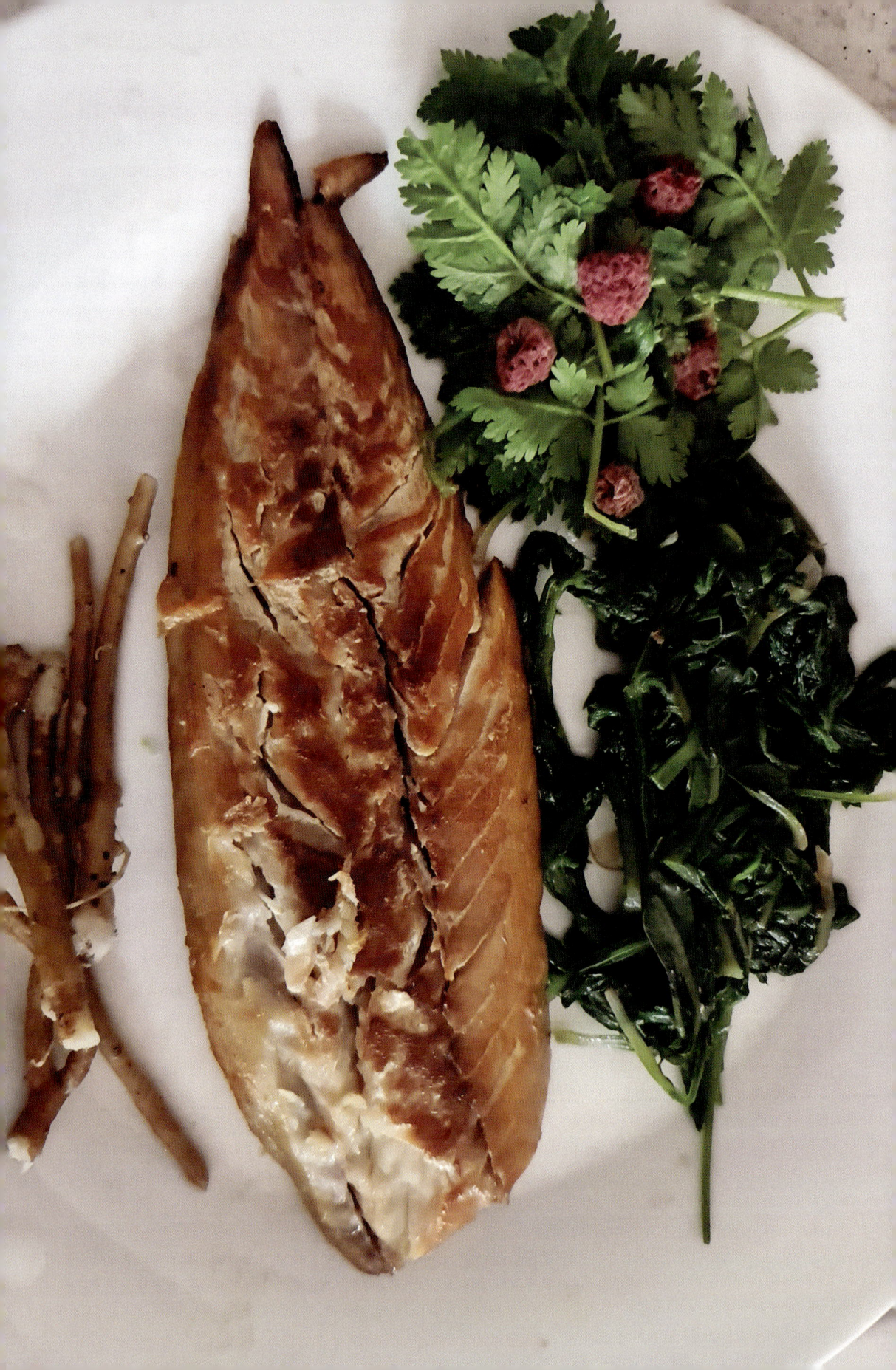

them home for dinner. Dinner is leftover venison, rosehip and wild garlic stew with the nettles airfried on top. Really delicious.

Day 8

I wake up having to rush to the toilet again with really loose bowels. I'm tired. I want to spend today indoors. It's only day 8. I know that my microbiome could take a while to adjust so I'll leave it at that. It's a day off, and I spend the day relaxing and cozying up. I graze on dried berries, apples and a couple of boiled eggs all day. My activities are very sedentary and restful. I sleep well.

Day 9

It's Easter Sunday and I perk up. Rest days are so important, and as my energy comes back so does my appetite. I've planned a bit of a feast. It's a celebration day, and with all days that I have in my calendar as celebration days I eat good food. But this year it can't involve chocolate.

I'm a dedicated chocoholic. I'm quite emotionally attached to chocolate and how it makes me feel. There's something wholesome once in a while not to have the usual treats and to mix it up. But this isn't mixing up, it's what I have available.

I recreate the chestnut on hazelnut flan base that Katy had on our day out to the seashore. I add stewed apples topped with a honey meringue. Well, that's just pudding but it's a welcome treat.

Also I'm having another day off and relaxing well, with time to go out again but with none of the pressures of day-to-day work. There's a few leaves of wild garlic left in the fridge when I go out to get dandelion roots and leaves. This time it's more of a gentle walk than a dedicated march to a spot for plants.

I have wild boar chops, which are becoming a firm favourite because they are so delicious. I dry fry the wild garlic and air fry some nettles. This combined with the pudding makes a fitting feast for a celebration day, and I'm all pleased with myself that I manage to make such a lovely meal in the middle of this experiment.

In the evening I settle down to watch a film and relax well before going to bed.

Day 10

I wake up having to rush to the toilet again. I assume this is down to the richness of the food from yesterday and my microbiome adjusting accordingly. I'll leave it at that and continue with my day.

Foraged Condiments

I've got good energy today. I decide to make something slightly different. I take the smoked mackerel and fashion it into fish cakes with an egg and chestnut flour plus sorrel and cleavers. I make a simple nettle purée sauce. I pan fry some woodrush and make a plantain and dandelion leaf salad with blaeberry vinegar. And one tiny pignut that I find. Pudding, despite this morning, is the leftover stewed apple and honey meringue tart.

I relax into the evening with a couple of fresh organic apples for snacking on.

Day 11

It's another day out, and Katy and I go along the old railway line. I show her where I have been picking from, and we move further and deeper into the woods. We both want to have enough for our dinner.

I'm really starting to feel immersed in this project, and I can sense the season changing more than I normally would. This is exciting as I feel myself tuning in more to the change of the season and the growth of the plants that I see every year. I've lived in this area for over 10 years and I know these plants really well.

This year is slightly different as I wait in anticipation for them to be big enough to add to my diet on a daily basis. I've eaten plenty of wild food and really enjoy the flavours, but they're normally something I add as a condiment, as sauces or a salad – a twist in a cocktail for the weekend.

This isn't playing anymore. But I'm starting to feel quite grounded in where my food is coming from and my own ability to gather enough food to feel sated.

We gather some more fresh nettle tops and some sorrel, a few young rosebay willowherb shoots, some dandelion leaves and a couple of gorse flowers. We collect enough for our dinner today and enough for Katy to put some in the fridge. Spring is a little bit further behind where she lives, so a bit of stockpiling is necessary.

I start to think about how with gardening we clip and prune but do not reflect on our impact. It's the same with what we are taking right now. I consider how we manage our environment, whether that be a small garden or a big estate, about how humans have shaped our environment and played a role and what we are living in now. I worry about our responsibilities for future generations and how our ancestors would have been doing the same thing I'm doing now.

I've also started to notice that my senses of smell and taste appear to be heightened. Is this because I'm not eating processed food? I don't eat much of it anyway. I'm not drinking alcohol, so has that cleaned up my body? I'm not taking sugars and hardly any carbohydrates. Is it a combination of all of these factors?

I'm not sure what's causing all this, but it feels good. Other folk in the group are reporting this as well.

Day 12

It's another desk day and I don't go out foraging today. I use the last of the wild boar chops. Because I didn't collect extra for myself yesterday I have some dried plants in the cupboard. It's nettles and burdock. I hydrate them and add them to the wild boar chops.

I take Yarrow out for her usual walks around the block, and pick one dandelion flower. I add it to my meal, if only to brighten it up.

Day 13

I wake up again with diarrhoea but continue with the day. It's another desk day.

I receive an unexpected parcel through the post. The lovely Lisa from Edulis Wild Food has sent me a care package of sea spaghetti, chestnuts, acorns and walnuts. How kind is that! She knew that when we went out to get seaweed I couldn't find sea spaghetti and kindly sent us some in the post. I promptly put it in the freezer.

I have unsmoked mackerel fish cakes with the chestnut purée, cleavers, nettles and some fresh young rosebay willowherb shoots.

Day 14

I wake up again with the disrupted digestion and want to understand what's going on.

One of the great aspects of this project is the community of us all doing it together. We meet regularly on a Tuesday and Friday evening via videocall, share our experiences and support each other. Other people in the group have also had loose bowels, and it appears to be just adjusting to the new food and a change possibly in the microbiome.

So I contact Monica Wilde and speak to her about what's happening with my digestive tract.

I'm perimenopausal, and my GP had suggested to me to look at histamine for some of my symptoms. As a herbalist I deal with most of my own hormonal imbalances and the symptoms it can create. I'd worked on my nervous system with relaxing herbs and techniques to help bring it to a better place. So I considered histamine as something I should look at more deeply.

When talking to Mo and doing some research I realise I have been taking a lot of high-histamine foods in this diet to this point. So in order to test this theory and to help possibly alleviate any gastric issues I switch to a low histamine diet.

For years I've talked about the spring cleanse, and I'm here I am doing it. I find this exciting. It's time to stop talking about it and start doing it – I just didn't expect it to be like this. But I know what to do and get on with it.

I decide to be quiet for a while on social media. I do social media but I wouldn't say that I enjoy it, and I feel it's OK to take a break while I work out how to do my spring cleanse. The next few days I will stay quiet and work from home. My food is very simple and is mostly filled with the usual snacks and fresh apples.

Day 17

So I wake up full of energy and ready to go. I have eggs for breakfast but without the nettle seed. I eat fresh apples for lunch, and for dinner I have smoked mackerel on a bed of cooked dandelion leaves with boiled dandelion roots and a small salad of cleavers and dandelion leaves. It's a clinic day and it's full of videocalls helping folk. I feel good at the end of the day and settle easily into a relaxing evening. Sleep arrives well.

Day 18

It's another day out with Katy and the dogs. We travel out a bit closer to Katy's house on a quiet road I'm very familiar with. We both have good energy, and end up like a couple of young girls, excited and settled into our task.

It's become a joy, not a task. Plus now the plants are really starting to come up and there's a lot more for us to have for dinners. I always get excited to see the plants coming up in Spring – it's like seeing old friends again. We joyfully almost skip from plant to plant.

We take the dogs into some nearby woodland, and find wood sorrel coming up and even in flower. We nibble just a few. It's a delightful flavour, light and bright on the tongue. I find chickweed starting to come through and am delighted. Jack in the hedge is also making an appearance above ground.

I show Katy pignuts, and she finds her first one. It always makes folk smile when they get a pignut. It can be difficult. We gather enough for our dinners today and a few more days for Katy, but the difference is there are new plants to add to the plate now. I have smoked haddock with dry fried wild garlic leaves, boiled dandelion leaves and roots, and cleavers. Along with a Jack in the hedge leaf, common sorrel and chickweed salad.

Day 19

I wake up feeling great, and my digestion seems settled at last. Today I have to take a fair amount of foraged nettle tops into the Fish Shop in Ballater. This is the first time I've gone out somewhere with a task and not had any anxiety. The fish shop isn't open yet but there are a few people there trying items on the menu. It's a soft opening.

I see a few familiar faces. One friend in particular, Avril, rushes over and gives me a hug. She knows it's not been easy for me this last year. I feel very supported and loved. Thank you, Avril. I see Hollie who has started working at the fish shop, and we hug too.

It's a lovely way to start going back to work. My big win personally is not having any anxiety at all. I feel so good I decide to drive to Braemar and see how driving feels. It's fine, and I settle well this evening after a dinner of smoked mackerel, boiled dandelion leaves with cleavers, sweet cicely leaf salad and wild raspberry vinegar.

I should mention I haven't been draining away the water from boiling. I've been drinking it. My amazing Uncle Reg, 90, taught me this. Since learning from him I have been doing it with my boiled veg, so it made sense to continue with it.

Day 20

Today is a clinic date. I'm working for the CLAID (Covid, Lyme and Infectious Disease) herbal clinic at Napiers.

I've got a student today from the Heartwood programme at the National Institute of Medical Herbalists. She's a very sweet lady, kind and smart. She's actually an old patient of mine. As she walked out the door on her last appointment she said 'I'm going to train to become a herbalist, and I want to learn from you.' Here we are a few years later and she is there as a student. This makes me feel great, teaching the next generation of herbalists. I spend the day snacking and don't make a full meal.

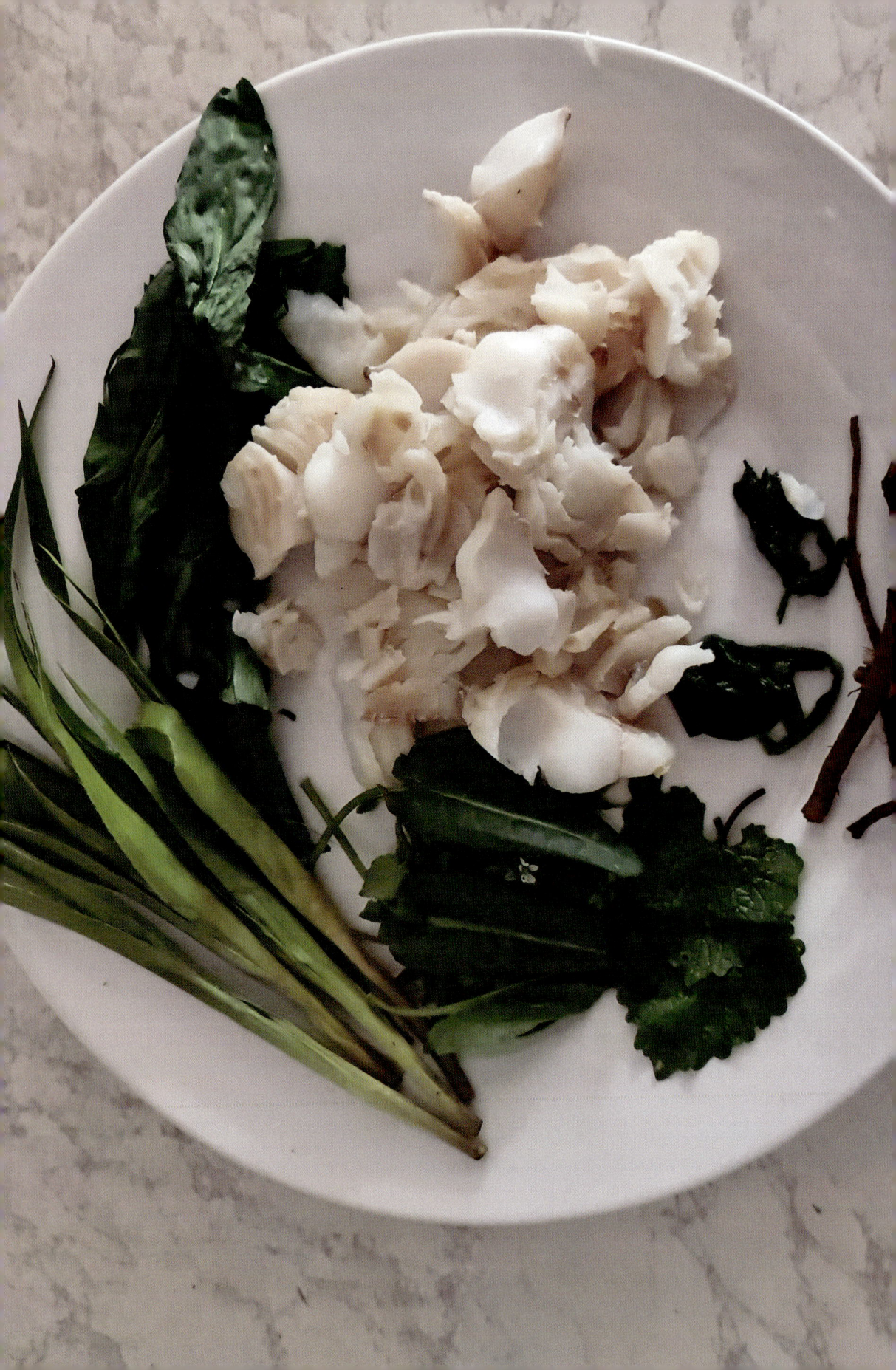

Day 21

I wake up feeling great again and with a new vigour. So I try some new recipes after going out and getting a few leaves. It's a bit of a paperwork day after yesterday, with patient notes and prescriptions to write up. Once that's done I get outside. I'm feeling completely on a roll with this. I feel great and settled.

I bake an apple with dried blaeberries, raspberries and chopped hazelnuts, with half a teaspoon of honey. It's really delicious. I'm not too sure why I haven't done this before. I pull out the sea spaghetti that Lisa sent, and pluck up the courage to try it. On top of the sea spaghetti I have baked cod with a rosehip purée and dried pan fried wild garlic, topped with some pickled wild garlic flower buds. It's a really delicious meal.

Day 22

Today I have my first walk back at The Fife Arms for a long time. I make sure I've got enough snacks with me and water. It's just two hours, but it can take your energy. It turns out to be a lovely couple who happened to work with gut biome and mental health, which makes for a really interesting walk. We talk loads. They haven't heard of the Wild Biome project, so I fill them in enthusiastically.

My energy is good, my mood is good and I go to home content. I have baked haddock with boiled dandelion roots and leaves with cleavers. I sprinkle it with a few dried sweet cicely leaves from a few days ago.

Day 23

One week to go. When did that happen? It feels like yesterday I started this project, which is testament to the rhythm I've got into. It's become second nature.

It's time to put on the blood sugar monitor and wear it for the last week of eating wild food and also the week after in which I'll go back to ordinary food. At this point I'm unsure of what I'll do. I know I want chocolate again, but how much of this experiment and project will I take into my day-to-day life afterwards? If it's improved my gut microbiome then I really don't want to undo that work. It's too early to think yet as I have a few days left.

Day 24

OK, now I know we're coming to an end I'm starting to dream of food and what my first meal will be. That means changing back to my usual methods. I'm getting food in, and although it's only been a few weeks I actually it this quite difficult to change my brain back into ordering food again.

Yes, I'm a creature of habit and don't like change. I'm quite perplexed as to what it is that I want to eat again. I'm a meat eater and I would say I've been craving beef. I'm craving chocolate hugely, and a few G&Ts wouldn't go amiss. My local chip shop will tell you I'm a regular visitor, but I don't feel that I should have something so heavy as my first meal.

It's a Monday and it's a really busy Monday. I have lots of emails to reply to and catch up on. It's snowing with some hail in between. So with a combination of a busy day and inclement weather I stay in.

It's smoked mackerel again with dried nettles, dried burdock, some chestnuts and rose hip purée for dinner.

Day 25

A rest day, but I'm feeling OK go for a long walk with Yarrow, to clear my head from yesterday's workload and to think about the changes that are about to occur. I don't pick anything and I just walk. I'm lucky to live in a place where walking is easy, and just outside my door there are several very nice walks.

I snack most of the day on a couple of boiled eggs and fresh apples.

Day 26

It's another day of collecting for the fish shop. The nettles have grown a lot in the last week, which makes my task easier. I bring in the nettles, take them to the kitchen, weigh them and go to leave. A few folk ask how it's going and how I'm feeling on the diet, and am I looking forward to finishing?

I have mixed feelings about this. I'm proud I have managed it, but until the results come through I won't know if it's helped my gut microbiome or not. I can say I have no anxiety, my mood is good and my energy is good. All are positive signs.

I go for a quick walk, looking for a few plants to take home. Yarrow stops at the gate. Her friend Teddy is in his garden, so I let her into the garden. Alison is there so we chat for a while, and she offers me some wild garlic from her garden. I have forgotten about this or I would have asked earlier. I'm delighted that I don't have to go very far today. I take up her offer, and I find a very good reason to go on to social media. A supportive and kind community are really important. We need a strong community.

Day 27

It's another clinic day. Today I struggle doing social media and decide to take a rest day. I get on with my usual household tasks and change the cupboard slightly in the kitchen in preparation for the change that's about to occur. Then I came up on the sofa. Me and Yarrow snuggle for an evening of lectures and then a film.

Day 28

Rest day.

Day 29

It's the last day of eating wild food. My supermarket order has arrived. Yes, it has chocolate in it. I'm excited and nervous on how my body is going to react. This diet has had an impact on my mental health and nervous system, and I don't want to move away from that.

Along with the usual snacks of dried berries and fresh organic apples my evening meal is a wild green omelette with cleavers, dandelion leaves, wild garlic with some woodrush, and a salad of dandelion leaves and flowering currant leaves.

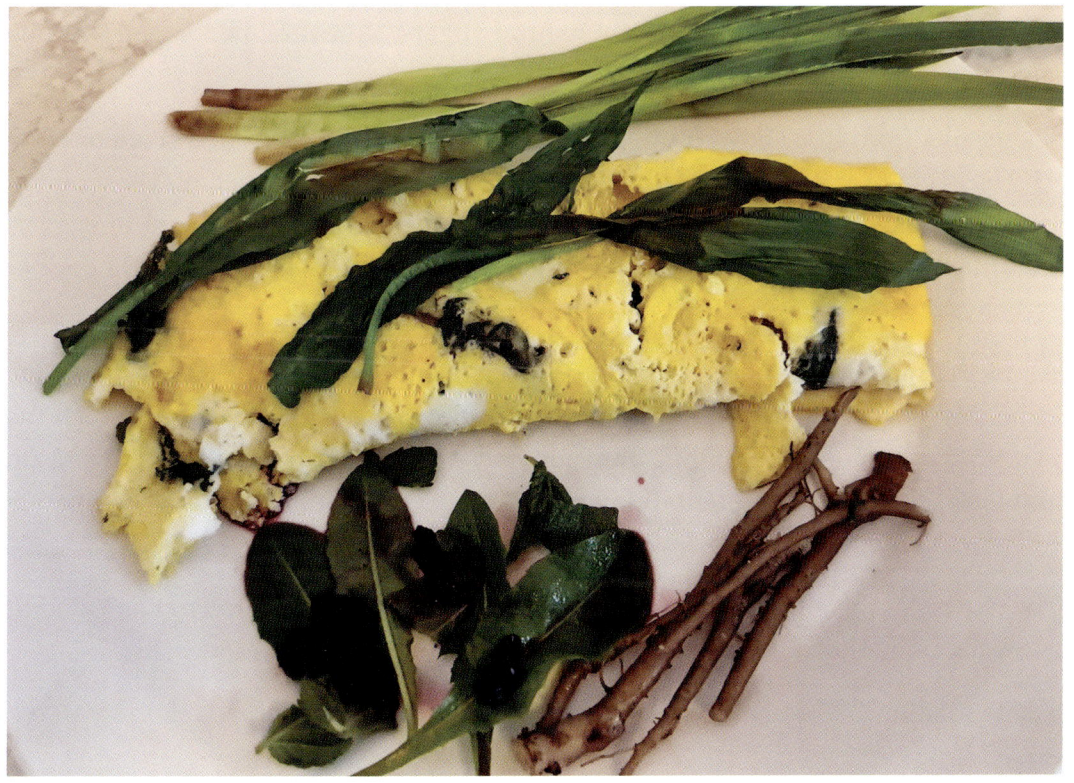

Day 30

I can eat whatever I want today, but first I have some tests to do. I have to collect a small stool sample for the gut microbiome test, and take two blood samples for nutrition markers and hormonal markers. Then I can have breakfast.

This is porridge with linseed, peanut butter and dried blaeberries. I have just a small portion. It's a lot of carbs in one go after not having many carbs for a month. It sits well. I then eat some chocolate, and it tastes divine. My first meal is mince and tatties with rosehip as the sauce, not tomatoes. It's really good and comforting.

Results

The results were so far have been interesting. Personally, I have not had the same level of anxiety again, and my digestion has improved. Since doing the diet I have eaten mostly organic food and avoided anything with preservatives in it. I sort of did this before, but now I'm quite strict.

I have included carbohydrates again, but not at the same level they were before. I've reduced my drinking of alcohol as this has an effect on the microbiome. Sugar eventually crept back in, but mostly natural sugars, unless refined sugar is in the chocolate bar.

The results from Zoe showed my gut bacteria had improved from a score of 69 to 93. The average at Zoe is 50. My blood sugar went down in the diet, maybe a bit too low sometimes. My cholesterol went up, I suspect owing to the amount of eggs as towards the end I wanted to include more fat to give more energy with the lack of carbohydrates.

All of the nutritional markers B12, magnesium and vitamin D3 stayed about the same. My hormones showed high levels of oestrogen at the beginning, which fits in with the perimenopause, but unfortunately I got the two blood tests mixed up and took the test at a different time in my cycle so the results cannot be compared. Inflammation markers went down.

The results for the group look very favourable for improving gut microbiome and as a low inflammation diet. The full results can be found at Monica's website:

The Wildbiome™ Project Results - Mo Wilde (monicawilde.com)

Bibliography

Barker, J. *The Medicinal Flora of Britain and Northwest Europe*. 2001. West Wickham, Kent. Winter Press.

Bartram, T. *Bartram's Encyclopedia of Herbal Medicine*. 1998. London. Robinson Publishers Ltd.

Beith, M. *A'Chraobh: The Tree*. 2000. Sutherland. No.19 Dornoch Studio.

Beith, M. *Healing Threads*. 2004. Edinburgh. Birlinn Ltd.

BHMA. *British Herbal Pharmacopoeia* 1983. 1999. Bournemouth. BHMA.

Bird, F. *The Forager's Kitchen*. 2013. London. CICO Books.

Brown, C. *A Year in a Scots Kitchen*. 1998. Glasgow. Neil Wilson Publishing Ltd.

Bruton-Seal, J. & Seal, M. *Hedgerow Medicine*. 2008. Ludlow. Merlin Unwin Books.

Bruton-Seal, J. & Seal, M. *Kitchen Medicine*. 2010. Ludlow. Merlin Unwin Books.

Bruton-Seal. J. & Seal, M. *The Herbalist's Bible*. 2014. Ludlow. Merlin Unwin Books.

Bruton-Seal, J. & Seal, M. *Wayside Medicine*. 2017. Ludlow. Merlin Unwin Books.

Buchan, D. *Folk Tradition and Folk Medicine in Scotland*. 1994. Edinburgh. Canongate Academic.

Child, J., Bertholle, L. & Beck, S. *Mastering the Art of French Cooking*. 2009. London. Penguin.

Clyne, D. *Gaelic Names for Flowers and Plants*. 1989. Furnace, Argyll. Cruisgean.

Darwin, J. *The Scots Herbal*. 1997. Edinburgh. Mercat Press.

Duke, J. *The Green Pharmacy*. 1997. Emmaus, PA. Rodale Press.

Ehrenreich, B. & English, D. *Witches, Midwives & Nurses*. 1972. Tacoma, WA. Lunaria Press.

Ganora, L. *Herbal Constituents*. 2021. Louisville, CO. HerbalChem Press.

Grieve, M. *A Modern Herbal*. 1931. London. Jonathan Cape Ltd.

Griggs, B. *Green Pharmacy*. 1981. London. Jill Norman & Hobhouse Ltd.

Grigson, G. *The Englishman's Flora*. 1958. London. Phoenix House.

Hatfield, H. *Hatfield's Herbal*. 2009. London. Penguin.

Hoffmann, D. *Medical Herbalism*. 2003. Rochester, VT. Healing Arts Press.

Hoffmann, D. *The Information Sourcebook of Herbal Medicine*. 1994. Freedom, CA. The Crossing Press.

Kenicer, G. *Scottish Plant Lore*. 2020. Edinburgh. Birlinn Ltd.

Kingston, R. *Ireland's Hidden Medicine*. 2021. Hilltop, Lewes. Aeon Books.

Leyel, C. & Hartley, O. *The Gentle Art of Cookery*. 1983. London. Chatto & Windus. The Hogarth Press.

Martin, M. *A Description of the Western Isles circa 1695*. 2018. Edinburgh. Birlinn Limited.

Martynoga, Fi. *A Handbook of Scotland's Wild Harvests*. 2012. Glasgow. Saraband.

McGarry, G. *Brighid's Healing*. 2005. Sutton Mallet. Green Magic.

Mességué, M. *Health Secrets of Plants and Herbs*. 1981. London. Pan Books Ltd.

Michael, P. *Edible Wild Plants and Herbs*. 2007. London. Grub Street.

Mills, S. & Bone, K. *Principles and Practices of Phytotherapy*. 2001. London. Churchill Livingstone.

Pengelly, A. *The Constituents of Medicinal Plants*. 2004. Wallingford, Oxfordshire. CABI.

Robertson, K. & O'Rawe, D. *Celtic Herbal Medicine*. 2020. Kildonan, Isle of Arran. The Scottish School of Herbal Medicine Ltd.

Sinclair, L. & Holohan, C. *Scotland's Wild Medicine*. 2021. Heal Scotland Books.

Wilde, M. *The Wilderness Cure*. 2022. London. Simon and Schuster UK.

Wright, J. *The Forager's Calendar*. 2019. London. Profile Books Ltd.

Index

A'chraobh: The Tree (Beith), 26
agriculture, 15
aiolis
   Jack by the hedge aioli, 139
   Wild garlic bud aioli, 139
allelopathy, 65
allicin, 104
5-alpha reductase, 80
American Pharmacopoeia, 100
Andersen, H.C., 70
antigin tonic, 172, 173
antiviral vermouth, 180, 181
Apiaceae family, 40
apple
   Apple and valerian flower chutney, 120, 121
   Elderberry jam, 130, 131
   Hawthorn ketchup, 153
   Rosebay willowherb flower jelly, 136, 137
   Rosehip ketchup, 154
   Sweet cicely and apple chutney, 124
   Wild raspberry jam, 132, 133
Autumn Equinox, 25

Beaton family, 11
beetroot and hogweed seed sauce, 156
Beith, M., 26, 32
Beltaine, 59
Bennett, Margaret, 35
Bennett, Martyn, 35
berry tonic, 174, 175
betulinic acid, 91
birch
   Birch bark salt, 151
   Pickled birch leaf, 162
   Silver birch, 91–3
bishops weed. *See* ground elder
bitters, 192
   Chocolate bitters, 193
   Douglas fir bitters, 194
   Hawthorn bitters, 195
   Orange bitters, 193
bogbean (*Menyanthes trifoliata*), 30–3
Book of Bald, 16
A Botanical Guide to Health (Coffin), 111
Botanologia (Salmon), 65
botulin, 91
bramble (*Rubus fruticosus*), 34–6
   Bramble syrup, 185
   Bramble vinegar, 159
   Pickled brambles, 163
   Plantain leaf and bramble chutney, 125
British Herbal Pharmacopoeia, 100
Brown, E., 63–4
Brugsch Papyrus, 16
Buchanan, F., 35

Cameron, J., 16
Campbell, T., 70
Carmichael, A., 111
Chaga chai, 166, 167
Chan, M., 23, 24
chocolate bitters, 193
chutneys
   Apple and valerian flower chutney, 120, 121
   Pear and dandelion root chutney, 122, 123
   Plantain leaf and bramble chutney, 125
   Sweet cicely and apple chutney, 124
Clachan stones, 27
coating
   Sweet cicely coating, 158
Coffin, A.I., 111
Coleridge, S.T., 91
Coles, W., 65
Colonna, F., 100
Compleat Herbal (Pechey), 65
connection, 21, 27
cowbane, 23
cow parsnip, 41
Culpeper, N., 40, 46, 65
cultivated food, 17–18

dandelion (*Taraxacum officinale*), 44–7
   Hawthorn bitters, 195
   Orange bitters, 193
   Pear and dandelion root chutney, 122, 123
   Spring pesto, 140
De Materia Medica (Dioscorides), 16
A Description of The Western Isles of Scotland (Martin), 16
Dioscorides, 16, 58, 100, 107, 111
dipping sauces, 117
   Hogweed seed dipping sauce, 118, 119
   Jack by the hedge, chilli and garlic dipping sauce, 117
Douglas fir bitters, 194

Ebers Papyrus, 16
Edwin Smith Papyrus, 16
elderberry (*Sambucus nigra*), 48–50
   Elderberry jam, 130, 131
   Elderberry rob, 171
   Elderberry vinegar, 159
   Ground elder cooking paste, 156
   Spring pesto, 140
   Wild garlic and elderberry vinegar dressing, 144
   Wild stuffing mix, 157
Emery, M., 36
endomycelium, 76
Evelyn, J., 49

The Family Herbal (Hill), 66
Fante, M., 24
fermented wild garlic, 128, 129

Foraged Condiments

ferments, 127
  Fermented wild garlic, 128, 129
  Traditional cabbage sauerkraut, 127
Fernie, W.T., 59, 69
fireweed jelly, 80
Flora Scotia (Lightfoot), 16
food
  cultivated, 17–18
  and medicine, 15
  supply chains, 197, 199–200
  sustainability, 199–200
foraged vermouth, 178, 179
forager
  calendar, 25
  modern, 200
foraging, 12
  balancing work and forage, 207, 209
  to cooking, 202–3
  immersion in wild, 210–11
  joys of, 213
  legacy of foraging traditions, 15–17
  mindful, 205–6
  in Scotland, 14–15
  at seashore, 206–7
  spring, 203–4, 212–13
  for sustainability, 17–18, 201
  vital lesson, 23–24
  and weeding, 17–18
  wild foraging and survival, 203–4
  for wild garlic, 12–13

The Gaelic Names of Plants (Cameron), 16
Galenic Corpus (Galen), 16
Galen of Pergamon, 16, 58
garlic, wild (*Allium ursinum*), 102–4, 201
  Fermented wild garlic, 128, 129
  Hawthorn spiced sauce, 155
  Jack by the hedge, chilli and garlic dipping sauce, 117
  Mustard. *See* Jack in the hedge
  Nettle and hazelnut pesto, 141
  Olive oil and fermenting juice salad dressing, 143
  Spring pesto, 140
  Wild garlic and elderberry vinegar dressing, 144
  Wild garlic bud aioli, 139
  Wild garlic pesto, 142
gathering, 13–15
Gerard, J., 40, 53, 65, 79
glucosinolates, 65
Goris, A., 58
goutweed. *See* ground elder
Grieve, M., 35
ground elder (*Aegopodium podagraria*), 52–4
  Ground elder cooking paste, 156

Handbook of Scotland's Wild Harvests (Martynoga), 66
harvest, balancing, 205–6
hawthorn (*Crataegus* spp.), 56–60
  Hawthorn bitters, 195
  Hawthorn ketchup, 153
  Hawthorn spiced sauce, 155
  Hawthorn Turkish delight, 188, 189

hazelnuts, 14
  Birch bark salt, 151
  Nettle and hazelnut pesto, 141
  Plantain seed salt, 149
  Spring pesto, 140
  Wild garlic pesto, 142
Healing Threads (Beith), 32
heptalogue, 46
Herball (Gerard), 65, 79
Herbal Medicine (Weiss), 111
Herbal Simples (Fernie), 69
Hildegard of Bingen, 91
Hill, J., 66, 100
Hippocrates, 15, 16, 49
Hippocratic Corpus, 16
hogweed, common (*Heracleum sphondylium*), 38–42
  flower, 39
  medicinal properties, 41
  seed, 23
hogweed seed, 23, 41
  Beetroot and hogweed seed sauce, 156
  Hogweed seed dipping sauce, 118, 119
  Hogweed seed syrup, 183
hot drinks and rob
  Chaga chai, 166, 167
  Elderberry rob, 171
  Ivan chai, 168, 169
  Pine needle tea, 170
  Valerian hot chocolate, 165
hunting, 13–15

I Ching, 112
inulin, 46
Ivan chai, 80, 168, 169
Ivan's tea. *See* Ivan chai

Jack by the hedge (*Alliaria petiolata*), 62–6
  Jack by the hedge aioli, 139
  Jack by the hedge, chilli and garlic dipping sauce, 117
jams
  Elderberry jam, 130, 131
  Wild raspberry jam, 132, 133
jellies
  Rosebay willowherb flower jelly, 136, 137
  Rowan berry jelly, 134, 135
Jennings, Dr, 59
John, M., 31

Kahun Gynaecological Papyrus, 16
K'Eogh, J., 107
ketchups
  Hawthorn ketchup, 153
  Rosehip ketchup, 154

language and nature, 26–7
Leclerc, H., 33
LeSassier, W., 41
Lightfoot, J., 33, 35, 16, 49, 112
lime flowers
  Antigin tonic, 173

   Chocolate bitters, 193
   Douglas fir bitters, 194
   Foraged vermouth, 179
   Hawthorn bitters, 195
   Lime flower tonic, 176, 177
Linnaeus, C., 41
Liot, A., 58
London Medical Papyrus, 16

MacLeod, M., 31
Martin, M., 16, 70
Martynoga, F., 66
mindful foraging, 205–6
A Modern Herbal (Grieve), 11, 35
mother of the heart. *See* hawthorn
mountain ash. *See* rowan

Naturalis Historia (Pliny the Elder), 16
nature
   connecting with, 21–3
   language and, 26–7
nettle (*Urtica dioica*), 68–70, 114, 200
   harvest and community connections, 216
   Nettle and hazelnut pesto, 141
   Nettle seed gomasio, 147
   Spring pesto, 140
   Wild stuffing mix, 157

oatcakes, 199
olive oil
   Hogweed seed dipping sauce, 118, 119
   Jack in the hedge, chilli and garlic dipping sauce, 117
   Nettle and hazelnut pesto, 141
   Olive oil and fermenting juice salad dressing, 143
   Spring pesto, 140
   Wild garlic pesto, 142
   Yarrow flower salad dressing, 145
oral traditions, 24–5
orange bitters, 193

Parkinson, J., 100
Pechey, J., 65, 87, 100
pestos
   Nettle and hazelnut pesto, 141
   Spring pesto, 140
   Wild garlic pesto, 142
Peters, E., 20
Pharmacie Galénique (Goris and Liot), 58–9
pharmacognosy, 99–100
phenology, 18–20
pickles
   Pickled birch leaf, 162
   Pickled brambles, 163
   Pickled rowan berries, 163
   Pickled wild raspberries, 161
pine
   cones, 87
   Pine needle tea, 87, 170
   Pine pollen sugar, 152
   resin, 87

   Scots pine, 86–8
pineapple mayweed (*Matricaria discoidea*), 72, 73
   Foraged vermouth, 179
   Pineapple mayweed infused vodka, 186, 187
   Pineapple mayweed syrup, 182, 183
   Pineapple mayweed Turkish delight, 191
pioneer plant, 79
plant
   and alphabet, 26
   identification, 23–4
plantain (*Plantago lanceolata* and *P. major*), 74–6
   Plantain leaf and bramble chutney, 125
   Plantain seed salt, 149
Pliny the Elder, 16, 75
Provision for the Poor in time of Dearth and Scarcity (Sibbald), 16, 65
'The Pursuit of Diarmuid and Gráinne', 83
pycnogenol, 88

Ramesseum Medical Papyri, 16
ramsons. *See* garlic, wild
raspberry, wild (*Rubus idaeus*), 106–9
   Berry tonic, 174, 175
   Pickled wild raspberries, 161
   Wild raspberry jam, 132, 133
Rooney, M., 197
rosebay willowherb (*Chamerion angustifolium*), 78–81
   Rosebay willowherb flower jelly, 136, 137
   Rosebay willow leaves, Ivan chai, 168, 169
rosehip
   Foraged vermouth, 179
   Ketchup, 154
   Syrup, 179, 185
rose tonic, 175
rowan (*Sorbus aucuparia*), 82–4
   Pickled rowan berries, 163
   Rowan berry jelly, 134, 135
   Rowan berry syrup, 184

Saint Gerard of Toul, 53
salad dressings
   Olive oil and fermenting juice salad dressing, 143
   Wild garlic and elderberry vinegar dressing, 144
   Yarrow flower salad dressing, 145
salicylates, 91
Salmon, W., 65
salts
   Birch bark salt, 151
   Nettle seed gomasio, 147
   Plantain seed salt, 149
   Seaweed salt, 149
salvestrols, 107
saponins, 91
sauces, stuffings and coating
   Beetroot and hogweed seed sauce, 156
   Ground elder cooking paste, 156
   Hawthorn spiced sauce, 155
   Sweet cicely coating, 158
   Wild stuffing mix, 157
Scotland
   foraging, 14–15

oral traditions and preservation of knowledge, 24–5
traditional medicine, 24
Scots pine (*Pinus sylvestris*), 86–8
The Scottish Naturalist (Buchanan), 35
seasonal changes, 25
and sensory awareness, 18–20
seaweed salt, 149
Sibbald, R., 16, 65
silver birch (*Betula pendula*), 90–3
sinigrin, 65
snowy waxcap mushroom, 76
spring
cleanse and gut health, 211–12
foraging, 212–13
Spring Equinox, 25
Spring pesto, 140
stories, 26–7
sugar
Pine pollen sugar, 152
Summer Solstice, 25
sustainable gathering, 205–6
sweet cicely (*Myrrhis odorata*), 94–6
Sweet cicely and apple chutney, 124
Sweet cicely coating, 158
Sylva (Evelyn), 49
synergy, 58
syrups
Bramble syrup, 185
Hogweed seed syrup, 183
Pineapple mayweed infused vodka, 186, 187
Pineapple mayweed syrup, 182, 183
Rosehip syrup, 185
Rowan berry syrup, 184

Tabernaemontanus, 53
tannins, 107
tonic waters
Antigin tonic, 172, 173
Berry tonic, 174, 175
Lime flower tonic, 176, 177
Rose tonic, 175
traditional cabbage sauerkraut, 127
Turkish delights
Hawthorn Turkish delight, 188, 189
Pineapple mayweed Turkish delight, 191
Turner, W., 41

Umbelliferae family. *See* Apiaceae family

valerian (*Valeriana officinalis*), 98–101
Apple and valerian flower chutney, 120, 121
Valerian hot chocolate, 165
Valerian, or The Virtues of That Root in Nervous Disorders (Hill), 100
vermouths. *See also* tonic waters

Antiviral vermouth, 180, 181
Foraged vermouth, 178, 179
Vicks VapoRub, 87
vinegars
Bramble vinegar, 159
Elderberry vinegar, 159

weeding, 17–18
Weiss, R., 111
The Wildbiome™ Project Results, 218
wild diet/food
adapting to, 199
wild food challenge, 199
wild food diary, 197–218
Wilde, M., 197, 211
The Wilderness Cure (Wilde), 197
wild food experiment, 197–218
balancing harvest, 205–6
balancing work and forage, 207, 209
coping with unexpected in foraging experiment, 204–5
cravings and transition, 215–16
culinary creativity and wellness, 215
day of new flavours, 209–10
day of reflection, 216
Easter feast and celebrations, 209
ethics of sustainable gathering, 205–6
final day of wild food, 217
first meal after wild food experiment, 218
foraging at seashore, 206–7
foraging to cooking, 202–3
fresh foods and productive work, 212
joys of foraging, 213
mindful foraging, 205–6
nettle harvest and community connections, 216
passing on knowledge, 213
preparing for, 202
refreshing walk and connection with knowledge, 215
rest day, 209, 217
results, 218
simple meals and reflective moments, 211
spring cleanse and gut health, 211–12
spring foraging, 203–4, 212–13
wild foraging, 203–4, 210–11
wild stuffing mix, 157
Williams, M., 40
Winston, D., 70
Winter Solstice, 25
Wood, M., 41

yarrow (*Achillea millefolium*), 110–13
Antiviral vermouth, 180, 181
Chocolate bitters, 193
Douglas fir bitters, 194
Foraged vermouth, 178, 179
Orange bitters, 193
Yarrow flower salad dressing, 145